Healing What's Within is the book for th[...]gh to risk becoming acquainted with them[...]. And in Chuck DeGroat we have a guide[...]

CURT THOMPSON, MD, psychiatrist and autho[...] *...per Place* and *The Soul of Shame*

This book is a beautiful resource shaped not only by Chuck's clinical expertise and pastoral heart but also by his own hard-earned lived experience.

AUNDI KOLBER, MA, LPC, therapist and author of *Try Softer* and *Strong like Water*

Healing What's Within invites you to address the paths and voices that have taken you away from your true home and reorients you to what is the delectable delight you were meant to know as shalom.

DAN B. ALLENDER, PhD, professor of counseling psychology and founding president, The Seattle School of Theology and Psychology

I could pick so many words in *Healing What's Within* that ministered to my soul. But I choose just two now: *redemptive remembering.* Those healing words gently guided me as Chuck reminded me of how our extraordinarily kind and loving God *is looking for me.*

LAURA BARRINGER, advocate and coauthor of *A Church Called Tov* and *Pivot*

Drawing on his personal, pastoral, and counseling experience, Chuck DeGroat offers a kind invitation toward emotional and spiritual healing, providing stories, practices, and resources to allow for whole-person engagement.

MANDY SMITH, pastor and author of *Unfettered* and *Confessions of an Amateur Saint*

In *Healing What's Within*, we are invited to acknowledge wounds, rediscover faith, and embark on a path of genuine restoration. This is a courageous and compassionate exploration of a path to great healing forged by God's pursuit.

JUSTIN S. HOLCOMB, Episcopal bishop, seminary professor, and author

With exceptional tenderness, breathtaking human stories, theological depth, and therapeutic insight comes *Healing What's Within*. Really, this manifesto of healing is like finding that wise sage you've been desperate to have a conversation with.

DAN WHITE JR., cofounder of The Kineo Center and author of *Love over Fear*

I find Chuck to be an effective healer based on a rare combination of practical wisdom, insightful empathy, and tender pastoral affection. All this shines through in *Healing What's Within*. I heartily recommend it.

BISHOP TODD HUNTER, Anglican bishop and author of *Deep Peace*

Healing What's Within is a practical guide on how to develop a holistic spirituality and practice that deals with real-world, real-person issues. This book is a gift to those who long for and thirst for righteousness.

MATT TEBBE, coauthor of *Having the Mind of Christ* and copastor at The Table, Indianapolis

Beyond making space for trauma, Chuck offers a healing path through it. Instead of seeing the Fall as God's rejection that activates our protective strategies, Chuck reminds us that God's connective pursuit is what heals the hurt within.

GEOFF HOLSCLAW, PhD, coauthor of *Does God Really Like Me?* and cohost of the *Attaching to God* podcast

In this beautifully gentle book, Chuck helps us to encounter a God who meets us in our most vulnerable places, not with harsh condemnation and punishment, but with compassion and curiosity, leading us toward healing the wounded places in our souls.

BEN STERNKE, cofounder of Gravity Commons, copastor at The Table, Indianapolis, and coauthor of *Having the Mind of Christ*

God's messengers come in many shapes, forms, and sizes, and I believe Chuck DeGroat is one of them. Here, his words wave a bright sword of truth, not swung menacingly to keep out but joyously to welcome in, calling with the tender voice of Jesus, "Here! Here is the way home!"

TARA M. OWENS, author of *Embracing the Body*, spiritual director, and founder of Anam Cara Ministries

While we are indeed fearfully and wonderfully made, we are often wounded, weary, and wandering. *Healing What's Within* supports our journey toward a holy wholeness.

CHRISTINA EDMONDSON, PhD, CEO and cofounder of Truth's Table Foundation; coauthor of *Truth's Table* and *Faithful Antiracism*

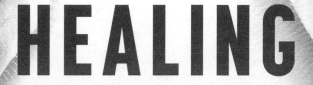

HEALING

Coming Home to Yourself—and to God—

WHAT'S

When You're Wounded, Weary & Wandering

WITHIN

CHUCK DEGROAT

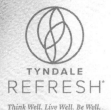

TYNDALE
REFRESH®

Think Well. Live Well. Be Well.

Visit Tyndale online at tyndale.com.

Visit Chuck at chuckdegroat.net.

Tyndale, Tyndale's quill logo, *Tyndale Refresh*, and the Tyndale Refresh logo are registered trademarks of Tyndale House Ministries. Tyndale Refresh is a nonfiction imprint of Tyndale House Publishers, Carol Stream, Illinois.

Healing What's Within: Coming Home to Yourself—and to God—When You're Wounded, Weary, and Wandering

Cover design by Lindsey Bergsma

Interior design by Laura Cruise

Published in association with Don Gates of the literary agency The Gates Group; www.the-gates-group.com.

For information about special discounts for bulk purchases, please contact Tyndale House Publishers at csresponse@tyndale.com, or call 1-855-277-9400.

The case examples in this book are fictional composites based on the author's professional interactions with hundreds of clients over the years. All names are invented, and any resemblance between these fictional characters and real people is coincidental.

Library of Congress Cataloging-in-Publication Data

A catalog record for this book is available from the Library of Congress.

ISBN 978-1-4964-8314-0

Printed in the United States of America

30	29	28	27	26	25	24
7	6	5	4	3	2	1

Contents

Foreword

I NEEDED *HEALING WHAT'S WITHIN* about twenty years ago, when the neglected fragments of my soul almost cut me from within.

To get some idea of my situation, picture a church with stained glass windows. If you look at them from the outside, those windows seem dull and unremarkable. Yet from the inside, as sunlight pours through them, they are spectacularly transformed. Each fragment of brightly colored glass glimmers and shines, dancing harmoniously with the others to illuminate the interior—a sanctuary that is warm, inviting, whole, *holy*.

Those stained glass windows illustrate how I presented myself back then—only in reverse. For years, I worked hard to maintain a calm, capable, and pleasing *exterior*. But internally, I battled chronic loneliness, anxiety, and pervasive self-doubt, often feeling sidelined in my own life. I felt unseen and disjointed, even as I worked to appear vibrant and put-together to others.

It was as if I lived as two different people: the capable Christian woman visible to the outside world, and the inner me, where painful emotions were walled off, buried, and pushed down.

I had excellent coping tactics to maintain this divide. I would rationalize or logic myself out of hard feelings, telling myself, *You have Jesus. You shouldn't feel this way. Focus on others.* When those mental gymnastics stopped working, I turned to numbing. I sought solace in binge-watching television, diving into the problems of others, or seeking comfort in food.

Then one day both strategies stopped working, and the untended shards of my soul burst to the surface in the form of a debilitating series of panic attacks.

I was a therapist and a doctoral student studying both psychology and theology. I sought genuinely to follow Jesus. Yet I had no clue how to take all that light I was working so hard to shine outwardly and redirect it to illuminate the fragments of my own soul. I had no clue that God longed for that light to radiate inside me too.

I didn't have the voice of my friend and spiritual brother, Chuck DeGroat, to guide me back then. But thankfully, I have it now. And so do you.

It takes an extraordinary person to courageously travel beyond these stubborn protective layers—the outer (often religious) armor of having it all together, the self-berating armor of shame and criticism, and the numbing armor of systematically checking out. It takes a brave person who—from that place beyond those defenses—turns back to help the rest of us find and heal what's broken and hurting within ourselves.

Chuck DeGroat is that person. And *Healing What's Within*

is the beautiful guide he's gifted us as we take this journey. Books like this aren't just written. They're lived, embodied, then revealed by someone who has traveled ahead and then stopped to illuminate the path for those of us still wandering. Chuck has already taught us to name and understand the reality of narcissism—not only in our leaders but also within ourselves. It's fitting, then, that he would now be the one to guide us on a journey of returning Home to ourselves.

Healing What's Within is more than a book—it's an encounter, an invitation, a mirror through which you will begin to see yourself. With fierce kindness and deep tenderness, Chuck skillfully redirects your gaze to the powerful questions God has been asking all along:

Where are you?
Who told you that it had to be this way?
Where have you taken your hunger?

You may feel vulnerable as you encounter God's loving presence through these questions. I did. But you won't feel shamed. Instead, you'll encounter a God who is patient, kind, and gentle, a God who sees, but never shames; who asks, but never manipulates; who invites, but never coerces. A God who seeks, above all else, to heal.

If you, like me, have exhausted yourself maintaining the facade of having it all together; if you've been harshly self-critical, judgmental, or shaming; if in desperation, you've numbed, avoided, or distracted yourself to your own or someone else's detriment, I am so glad you are here. I'm so grateful that you get to take this journey inward with my friend Chuck's kindness, compassion, and hard-earned wisdom as your guide.

Linger as you read these pages. Take your time. This is such good, important work, this endeavor to discover and sustain a Home within yourself—a beautiful inner sanctuary, where the stained glass windows of your soul are radiant in both directions.

Dr. Alison Cook
Therapist, coauthor of Boundaries for Your Soul, *author of* I Shouldn't Feel This Way, *and host of* The Best of You *podcast*

THE BETTER STORY

We who follow Jesus are working in wounds,
working with wounds, and working through wounds.
WILLIE JAMES JENNINGS

TWENTY YEARS AGO, I WAS FIRED.

After six years as a pastor on staff at the church where my daughters were baptized, where deep friendships were formed, where I founded a counseling center, and where I walked people through the dark nights of their lives, I was thrust into my very own dark night.

If I were you, I'd want the dirty details. Why was I so unceremoniously fired? Who was to blame? What was the fallout?

This isn't that book.

Because the thing is, what happened *to* me isn't as important as what happened *within* me in those months and years after. On the outside, I appeared resilient; people told me I was "strong," that I seemed to be bearing it all well, even praising the way our family was able to graciously pivot and cobble together an income in the aftermath. It appeared that I took it all in stride: I was fine—*better*, even—for the experience.

But on the inside, I stewed and stormed, feeling a constant churn that left me with daily stomach pain and heartburn, simmering anger and searing shame. Vital and happy just months before, I now hardly recognized myself, so consumed was I by the injustice of it all. I'd write and delete emails by the dozen, the rage welling up within me in great waves. I'd obsess about disappointing others, terrified of being rejected again. I'd nurse a constant nagging anxiety. In an attempt to rebuild my sense of worth, I'd work to the point of exhaustion.

I wondered: Were people quietly talking about me behind the scenes? Would the shame follow me wherever I worked or moved to? Did anyone care about what really happened? Was there anyone who'd have my back?

I felt utterly alone.

Overwhelmed by the deafening silence of so many people I had once considered friends, fear swallowed me—fear that I'd run into a leader from the church at a grocery store, fear that those who fired me would sabotage my chances for future jobs, even fear that I would be caught in the truth that maybe I wasn't as fine as I appeared. I did all that I could to ignore the festering wound growing within me.

And yet it continued to chafe.

For five years, I couldn't admit my overwhelm, my powerlessness, my loneliness. Our family moved to a neighboring town, I worked several jobs, I kept myself busy trying to keep it all together, trying to keep the pain of my loss away. The mostly unprocessed shame, anger, and grief continued to simmer within, my body tense and vigilant, defenses always up, fearing I'd again be hurt. "Something deep inside of you has already tightened up," Henri Nouwen once wrote, musing on our tendency to self-protect. "'Watch out, plan your tactics, and hold your weapons in readiness.'"[1] And indeed, my body was postured for the possibility of more pain. Insulated with activity and thick layers of self-protective defenses, I lived chronically disconnected from any real source of care or love.

I wasn't myself, and somewhere deep down, I knew it.

• • •

We're all prone to do this, no matter the extent of harm or hurt. We toss and turn at night, remembering and even rehearsing what happened over and over again, its pain palpable. The storms within churn constantly. The thick fog doesn't let the light through. We may go for months or years fixated on the past, even trying to rectify the wrong—and then, we learn the survival skills to get by.

In our effort to pursue justice for what happened *to* us, we begin to hinder any chance at healing what's within. We cope alone, in isolation. We ignore our pain. We suppress our agonizing emotions. We disregard core needs. We distance ourselves from others. We normalize our grumpiness and our shame, our lonely and abandoned feelings, our numerous numbing tactics, our simmering anger. We normalize distracting ourselves from the everyday ache that haunts us, content to scroll through our phones with buzzing envy, looking for some dopamine hit of pseudo connection. Eventually, we lose touch with ourselves. We succumb to a sense of dulled desire. We stop noticing that we feel out of sorts a lot of the time. Even our faith feels dry, relegated to simply going through the motions.

There are a hundred reasons why we choose to cope instead of confront this ache—this *disconnection*—inside us. In the wake of being fired, I rehearsed a litany of reasons why I was just fine, why I, of all people, didn't need help, didn't need to reach out for care. I've said some of them, and in my counseling practice, I've heard them all:

- Far worse things have happened to others.
- It's not as bad as I think.
- I don't have time for arduous introspection.
- I can deal with this on my own.
- I just need to be more positive.
- God wants me to focus on others, not myself.
- I'm just the way I am. It's my personality.
- People don't really change.
- I'm strong, and I've gotten through harder things.
- If I look into my past, I'll just open up a whole can of worms.

Left unchecked, this inner sense of alienation eats away at the core of who we are, wreaking havoc on our relationships with others and with God. At worst, it's *traumatic* to our hearts, bodies, and souls, leaving behind a hidden wound that can't heal without intentional care.

Yes, it can be traumatic, indeed. "Trauma is perhaps the most avoided, ignored, belittled, denied, misunderstood, and untreated cause of human suffering," psychologist Peter A. Levine writes.[2] And while the word *traumatic* is undoubtedly misused by those who call their team's Super Bowl loss or a phone dropped in the toilet traumatic, many of us who do the work of caring for souls believe that we don't name the ill effects of trauma in our lives quite enough. Because at the heart of trauma lies profound disconnection.

And disconnection is a story as old as time itself.

●　●　●

I still remember the dark and damp church classroom on Long Island, New York, where I'd see the epic Bible stories come to life on flannel board. The vivid greens, ocean blues, and brilliant yellows provided the landscape backdrop to flannel figures of the great heroes of Scripture. Noah smiling atop his boat (even as people drown in the waters below). Abraham brimming with pride before his son (even as his knife lies nearby). Ruth and Naomi cheerfully walking side by side (even as the stench of death lingers). Adam and Eve standing together, rosy-cheeked grins on their faces, grass skirts covering their privates (even as they vigilantly scan to see if God is coming). All flannelgraph images that fail to convey just how traumatic a life exiled from God and ourselves can be.

The Bible may begin in connection, just like your story and mine, but the tides quickly turn; by the third chapter, rupture manifests in shame and exile—a profound disconnection. The full account of Genesis 3 is too brutal to fit into that flannel-graph faith; Adam and Eve may be filled with shame and hidden behind fig leaves according to the ancient story, but on the flannel board they're posing with smiles on their faces, a snake grinning nearby.

What's more, I was taught that Adam and Eve eating the fruit of the tree and going into hiding was the *central* story of how everything went wrong in the world, even what was wrong with me to the core. And God's anger proves it.

Where are you? God asks, fuming from the ears.

Who told you? God demands to know, finger pointed at Adam and Eve.

Have you eaten from the tree? God compels them to answer, forcing them—and us—from the Garden forever.

The heading at the top of that third chapter of Scripture— "The Fall."

Indeed, we return to the story time and again because it resonates so deeply with what's within us, with *our* story, even who we suppose God is. It's a story that begins in intimate union and communion but too quickly turns to shame and alienation. It's a story of disconnection from ourselves, disconnection from each other, disconnection from our bodies, disconnection from God. The serpent's lie inflicts a wound, shattering trust and manifesting in a frantic search for a self-remedy in the fruit of the tree. This primal wound—this traumatic estrangement—continues to whisper within us the awful lie that God can't be trusted, that we're on our own, that our only hope is in grasping for the fruit, the enticing elixir that will quell the ache.[3] Yet as a longtime pastor and therapist—one who knows too well how such trauma can pervade a life—I've learned to read the story in Genesis 3 through a different lens. Yes, it's a story that reveals how we cope in ways that self-protect and sabotage. Yes, it's a story that reveals how we experience profound disconnection—with each other, with God, even with ourselves. Flannel boards can't cover up the facts.

But what if it is also a better story than we've been told, a story that shows us how we can acknowledge what's happened to us *while also* compassionately healing the wounds left behind? What if God's response to us is, in fact, kinder than we imagined?

Even as Adam and Eve are doused in shame, riddled with anxiety, and hidden behind fig leaves, God shows up in compassion and with curiosity, reconnecting even amidst the radical rupture, his voice a homing beacon. And the questions God poses hold the possibility for healing what's within us, for us to become ourselves again.

> *Where are you?* God asks with heartache, longing to
> find us.

Who told you? God asks with compassion, curiously
pursuing the story.

Have you eaten from the tree? God asks with gentleness,
tenderly bringing our eyes to where we've chosen
to cope—to numb, to soothe, to avoid—instead of
abiding in his care and compassion.

Indeed, that's a much better story—a more hopeful story
than the flannel boards ever revealed. If we dared to read it this
way, perhaps we'd reimagine a better heading than "The Fall" at
the top of the chapter—"God Longs for Us Even When We're
Lost." Or perhaps more simply, "Found."

You see, these core questions provide a path to our true healing. Not a surface-level healing that looks good on the outside,
but the healing of each of our souls, the deepest place within us.
These questions invite us to come home to ourselves when we're
wounded, weary, and wandering. As God says later through the
prophet Isaiah, even after Israel suffers its own profound trauma
and engages its own addictive strategies, "In returning and rest
is your salvation" (Isaiah 30:15).

•   •   •

In this book, we'll take these three questions, one by one, in
three parts, framing our journey together, our path to greater
healing forged by God's pursuit. As you're asked to attend to
the healing within you, you'll learn how to consider your own

wounds, to acknowledge the possibility of a disconnection within that is keeping you stuck and blocking the path to joy and flourishing. You'll then be invited to discover real rest and renewal as you reconnect with God, others, and yourself.

At the end of each chapter, you'll find additional resources, reflection questions, and next steps to practice. As you read, some of what I say may stir discomfort or raise questions, prompting a bit of internal resistance or even some confusion. But, as you are able, continue on. Remain curious. Come home to yourself and to God, and to a conversation within that your heart has needed for a long, long time.

God's kindness meets us right where we are, and God wants us to become curious about what's happening within, in our "inmost being" (Proverbs 20:27). "Trauma is not what happens to us, but what we hold inside in the absence of an empathetic witness," physician and trauma expert Gabor Maté writes.[4] God longs to be *your* empathetic witness, to attend to the wounds within you, to reconnect with you, to help you return to yourself. He has—quite literally—designed you to be known.

I get it if you're just not sure. Maybe you've been languishing in disconnection for so long that your desire is dulled. Maybe numbing is easier. Maybe this just feels too complicated. For moments like this, the wise novelist and nonfiction writer Anne Lamott has some modest advice. She counsels you to offer up to God a one-word prayer: "Help!" Lamott says that this is the simplest and most authentic prayer you can pray.[5] For a long and lonely season, it was the only real prayer I could muster.

Yes, it may feel like too much. It may even feel like it's too late. You may look back over the years, wondering where the time has gone. You may even look at some of the hurt you've endured and inflicted, wondering whether it's worth crying out for help. Whether it's worth going on this journey.

It's worth it. You're worth it.

PART 1

WHERE

Coming Home to Ourselves, Befriending Our Pain,

ARE

and Attending to Its Imprint Within

YOU?

WHERE AM I?

Awakening to Our Disconnection

*We all long for [Eden], and we are constantly glimpsing it:
our whole nature at its best and least corrupted, its gentlest
and most humane, is still soaked with the sense of "exile."*

J. R. R. TOLKIEN

"I'm just not myself," Rebekah tells me, grabbing a pillow on my office couch and pulling it toward her body. By all accounts, she should be happy. Or so she thinks. Rebekah and her husband live with their three young children in a newer home, they drive nice cars, and they take fun family vacations. She serves as a deacon at a church they love. She is the first person people call for parenting or budgeting tips, the first person people want to talk to at social functions. She is living the life she dreamed of, the life her teenage self thought she wanted.

Except, somehow, it doesn't feel like the dream she thought it would. "I should be grateful," she says, breaking eye contact with me for a moment as she looks out my window, her head shaking no, her face revealing hints of disgust. She tells me that when she scrolls through social media, she feels a vague ache as she clicks on photos of other women her age—some who've started businesses, others who've written a book or refinished a dresser or gone back to school for a graduate degree. Scrolling is soothing, for a time, but it eventually leaves her even more dissatisfied.

For a while, she tried to make sense of her discontentment through the latest personality tests and various self-help tools. She couldn't pinpoint when it had happened; she just knew she'd lost a sense of vitality and hope. Did she need therapy? A spiritual director? Maybe just a few days by herself? She wasn't sure. But she longed to find her way back home, to herself, to God, to a life of fullness and flourishing. "This is all just *so* typical of your Enneagram type," a friend insisted, handing her a new book to read. "I wouldn't worry about it. Just try to be more present. Start a gratitude journal or something!"[1] But her friend's advice didn't help, and the ache didn't abate. By day, the kids' routines would keep her busy—until that hour when the house would be completely quiet, the two oldest at school and the youngest napping. In the quiet her intrusive and often self-critical thoughts would get loudest, muted only with a bit too much food or drink in the evenings.

Unable to put her finger on the root of the void she felt, she doubled down, committed to embodying the perfect picture of her life she had sold to the world. She signed up for more events at church; she posted more pictures of her family on Instagram, all smiles and adventure; she picked up a couple more self-improvement books for her nightstand, just for good measure.

But in the therapy room with me, the facade breaks, if only

for an instant. Showing me a picture of her daughters, she tears up. "They're everything to me, and yet a part of me wants to disappear from the world. What kind of mom would think that?" Rebekah feels completely lost, unable to enjoy the life she had so carefully curated, overshadowed by sinking shame: What is wrong with her that this isn't enough? And what does it mean about *her* worth as a mom, as a wife, as a woman?

East of Eden

Perhaps you, like Rebekah, feel like something is missing or off within you or your relationships. Maybe you, like so many of us, have scrolled in search of it, or self-soothed in ways that elicit shame. You've looked for it in the gym. Or in a bit of flirtation with a coworker. Or perhaps the wearying search for it has left you hopeless, resigned to never finding what you'd hoped for. Your heart aches as you recall a time when you felt more alive, connected, and free. *Where am I?* you wonder. *And how did I get here?*

We're tossed amidst the storms of life and mired in the fog, and yet we've been conditioned to ignore our struggle, trained to smile and say, "Everything's fine." I've long wondered if the sanitized flannelgraph storytelling of our youth subtly communicated to our souls that we, too, need to button ourselves up, gloss over the hard stuff, and pretend we're living our best life in Eden, even when we're still faced with the heartache of exile.

Too often, we're sold cheap, three-step plans to the happy life, asked to believe in the power of positive thinking rather than invited to pray potent laments. Not long ago I sat for a week of intensive therapy with Jeff and Johanna, a couple who'd birthed a stillborn baby years before. They'd known for a couple of weeks that their daughter had died in utero before Johanna went into labor. "I wanted to scream," she said. "It felt like God was playing a cruel joke on us." But the hospital chaplain who visited them wanted to tidy up the story, offering a biblical rejoinder: "Rejoice always, pray without ceasing, in everything give thanks" (1 Thessalonians 5:16-18, NASB). Soon after, their pastor reiterated this, even telling them that God orchestrated all of this for their good.

After her husband, Jeff, heard this advice, he told me that he "walked away feeling a bit crazy, like, I couldn't be angry, I had to be grateful, even amidst what felt like a senseless death." The couple couldn't bear the disorientation, the vast canyon of ache between the pastor's answer and their reality. So their pain went underground. Johanna never did scream. Instead, she shut herself off from her honest emotions, relegating her heartache to the shadows, believing this to be the way of faith.

Neither one allowed themselves to feel grief or anger for a decade. Jeff became a workaholic, busy from the moment he got out of bed. Old addictions reared up as he became more and more cut off from himself and his own feelings, let alone Johanna's. She became emotionally numb, lost in a fog. Depression would wax and wane, but even on her best days, life seemed like an endless slog.

On the outside, Jeff and Johanna lived like a contented Christian couple, full participants in the life of their church.

But on the inside, utter disorientation and disconnection, even despair, ravaged whatever joy they had left.

I wonder what would've been different for Jeff and Johanna in the wake of their loss, or for Rebekah in the midst of her dissatisfaction, if instead of pushing away their pain they had learned to acknowledge it? What if God was inviting them to name how far from Eden they felt? How far from themselves they felt?

Navigating through the Fog

The morning temperature was 46 degrees, and the summer San Francisco fog was thick at 7 a.m. as I started my car for the drive to my therapist's office in Marin County. As I made my way north, I could hardly see the stoplights in front of me or the verdant greens of Golden Gate Park around me, an apt metaphor for how disoriented and disconnected from myself I felt in my second year back in pastoral ministry.

Now years after being fired, I lived in a new city and worked at a vibrant church that embraced me wholeheartedly, offering me every opportunity to thrive. But my body remembered what had happened six years prior. Within, a boiling cauldron of shame, self-doubt, fear, vigilance, anger, and unresolved grief threatened to bubble over. I could hardly remember the joy I once felt in the same work. And I worried about my growing reliance on ways of coping that only stirred the simmering pot within.

I wasn't myself, and I knew it. Like Rebekah, Jeff, and Johanna, I'd lost a sense of vitality. I was wandering in inner exile. I sought Eden in a new geography and in a fierce commitment to my work, proving myself indispensable and securing my sense of worth in the admiration of my colleagues and congregation. But the harder I tried, the further from home I felt. The further from myself I felt. And the God I'd commend to others in teachings and talks felt a million miles away too.

Every Tuesday morning, I'd navigate the labyrinthine drive north to my therapist's office, crossing the Golden Gate Bridge and winding my way through the Rainbow Tunnel, the fog finally dissipating before me to reveal Mount Tam in the distance. And this, too, felt like a metaphor for the slow work of returning to myself and rediscovering joy. It was on this foggy commute when I first heard the gentle whisper of God: "Where are you, Chuck?" The whisper was a homing beacon that awakened longing within me. I simply hadn't realized how exiled we could become from ourselves, from each other, and from God.

1,185 chapters

The Bible begins in Eden, a word that means "delight." The story begins in joy, in goodness, in connection. This is God's first home for us, and its memory abides deep within. But by chapter 3, disorientation, division, disorder, and disharmony make their appearance. We find a slithering serpent with lies on his tongue, his deceit dealing a blow to Adam and Eve's hearts, shattering trust and rupturing connection. Adam and Eve are enjoying union and communion with God and each other before the serpent slithers along.

His question is subtle, seeding their hearts with doubt and shame. "Did God really say, 'You must not eat from any tree in the garden'?" (Genesis 3:1). Imagine Adam and Eve's confusion. In a moment, the serpent twists the only script they have ever known, calling into question God's goodness, stirring doubt about their worth and belonging. *Can I trust God? Is God holding back something that I need, a fruit that will make my life better? Am I missing something?* As Sean Gladding writes, "The subtle serpent taps into our deepest anxiety as humans: the fear that what I have, no matter how good it may be, is not enough. The haunting suspicion that someone else has it better than me. That someone else *is* better than me. So, not only do I not have enough, I am not enough. I am less than."[2]

The serpent's lies shatter shalom and usher in traumatic disconnection, the disorder that captures headlines from then on:

Deceit
Shame
Blame-shifting
Enmity
Alienation
Murder
Adultery
Rape
Rivalry
Genocide
Heartache
Betrayal
Incest
Homelessness

And that's just in the first five books of the Bible!

This upheaval continues for 1,185 chapters before Jesus returns to make his ultimate home among us in Revelation 21 and 22. That's 1,185 chapters squeezed between two at the beginning and two at the end.

These 1,185 unavoidable chapters represent the story of our lives, the everyday ache you and I know east of Eden.

Through much of Scripture, the lived experience of God's people involved alienation and exile. Their strategies for coping were devastating.

> My people have committed two sins:
> They have forsaken me,
>   the spring of living water,
> and have dug their own cisterns,
>   broken cisterns that cannot hold water.
>
> JEREMIAH 2:13

And their heartache—every time they remembered home—was palpable:

> By the rivers of Babylon we sat and wept
>   when we remembered Zion.
>
> PSALM 137:1

This story places each of us in a tale of trauma and disconnection that no one is immune to.

Life amidst the 1,185 chapters we live within invites us to

reckon with the bitter realities we've avoided, including the depths of our disconnection from ourselves, from each other, and from God. Curt Thompson writes, "We are all born out of preludes of beauty and tragedy, each of us with our own ratio of both."[3] And while the beauty compels us to a life of restored relationship, the tragedy can't be ignored.

Attuning to the Healing Within

People who've seen me for soul care over the years know that I sometimes begin a session with a simple question: "Where do you find yourself today?" The question varies and shifts, but it's an echo of that very first question God asks in Genesis 3. It's an invitation to become curious about what's happening within. It's an invitation to return and retune, to awaken to the ancient whisper of love amidst the ache of alienation.

Some will tell me that it's been a good week, but after a bit of reflection, they recognize that they've merely been distracted from what's been simmering within. Others might share that they just don't know, that life has been a blur, that they're not entirely sure where they are or what's stirring inside of them. Still others have not had time to consider where they are because they've been attending to everyone and everything around them. Many of us don't know how lost we are. We've become habituated to a life of disconnection. We've developed a tragic case of amnesia, forgetting our original goodness and glory, far from home and without a map to guide us.

Indeed, it's true that we're disconnected, in part, because

we've walled ourselves off to what's happening within. But it's also the case that we've lost track of who we were created to be, our divine design, God's unique image within us with its possibility for fullness and flourishing in our lives.

And to understand how we've lost track of ourselves, we need to be reminded of where we began.

The Bible begins in connection, two chapters offering a glimpse of the glorious joy and intimacy God enjoyed with Adam and Eve. This life of goodness, this overflow of divine love, this is what we were made for, the imprint of God's image deeper than any traumatic imprint we'll ever encounter. To bear the image of God (Genesis 1:27) is to experience, at your core, an irrevocable inheritance of worth, belonging, and purpose.[4]

To live freely and fully from here is to know that you were created for deep *worth*—that you've been uniquely designed for dignity, that God delights in you, that you are enough, at your core.[5] It is to know that you were created for *belonging*—God the Trinity creates you for union and communion, for interdependence and intimacy with God, each other, and creation. And it is to know that you are created for *purpose*—stamped with God's image, which means that wherever you go, you go in the name of God, called by God, as an ambassador of God's shalom. This is your divine imprint, your deepest core, your impermeable identity, your irrevocable gift. This is the better and more hopeful story you've been designed for.

The Bible begins here, and this is where your story begins too. God has always longed to walk with you, even to make his home within you, closer to you than you are to yourself, as St. Augustine once said.[6] He's always wanted more for you than what you too often settle for. And our age-old dilemma is rooted in our inability to trust this goodness. It all goes back to that ancient tale.

"Every man has forgotten who he is," wrote the great English writer and philosopher G. K. Chesterton. "We are all under the same mental calamity; we have all forgotten our names. We have all forgotten what we really are."[7] Rebekah, Johanna, and Jeff forgot. And so did I. Sometimes the fog is so thick and the storms so intense that we lose our bearings. That's what the trauma of life within these 1,185 chapters can do.

But God goes looking, longing for us to come home.

Amidst Adam and Eve's ruptured relationship, God's first move is toward reconnection. "Where are you?" comes a voice, kind and longing.

At first glance, the question might seem silly to you. Of course, God knows where Adam and Eve are. But perhaps God wants them to recognize how hidden they are and how far they've ventured away. Perhaps God hopes they'll awaken with a new curiosity and maybe even a new hunger for home. And perhaps God wants the same for you.

God goes out looking for you, like any parent of one who is lost, like a compassionate father heartsick for his prodigal child. God's kind "Where are you?" invites you to pay attention to what's happening within, to attend to the storms that churn and the fog that dulls, disorienting and disconnecting you. And this requires courage. Too many of us grew up being taught to evade and avoid our ache, to be strong, to suffer alone. Too many of us are offered a flannelgraph faith story that minimizes the pain, that ignores our sense of alienation from ourselves and one another, that even cheapens the reality of God's compassion in our profound need. But God's "Where are you?" also invites each of us to remember who we are, at our core.

"The world is not served by those who are alienated from themselves and others, nor by those who in their pain bring pain to others," writes psychoanalyst James Hollis.[8] And yet many of us remain alienated for far too long. We lose track of how long because we're so busy, distracted, preoccupied, far from God and far from ourselves. We need to be reminded of a better story—that home is nearer than we imagine, that God is whispering from within, "Where are you?"

The Practice of Coming Home to Yourself

Many people admire Rebekah because she is so capable; as we talk, she recognizes that she'd been subtly trained in the ways of independence since she was very young. "No one told me I was on my own, but I knew I was," she says. Left alone for hours each day with younger siblings, she learned to cook, even do laundry. Later, she married a man who was aloof and distant himself, a recipe for a lonely life and the stirrings of despair. She feels adrift, longing for someone to really see her and, in so doing, help her find and validate her truest self.

Perhaps you, too, have been traveling a long, lonely road with too little presence and insufficient resources. You've been tugged by the old voices, taxed by too many obligations. You've pushed hard, trying to be strong. You've too often felt like you've had to keep it together, for yourself, for others who count on you.

You don't have to tread the impossible terrain alone anymore. It's time to long for more. It's time to unburden yourself. It's time to come home. To come to yourself.

What sounds a bit like a modern therapeutic cliché is actually ancient wisdom. St. Augustine of Hippo, a fourth-century North African bishop, wrote: "Do not go outward; return within yourself. In the inward man dwells truth."[9] And another revered saint of the twelfth century, Bernard of Clairvaux, wrote that God "restored to me the self that I had lost."[10] They heeded the homing beacon of God's kind voice calling them home, back to themselves. And so can you.

They, and many other saints, poets, psychologists, and sages through the centuries, believed that you and I get lost at times. The good life—even life in God—is already ours, but we go looking elsewhere, eventually losing not just God but ourselves in the process. "And where was I when I was seeking you?" Augustine writes. "You were before me, but I had gone away even from myself; nor did I find myself, how much less you!"[11]

Augustine's questions are ours, too. *Where am I?* We can go on for years ignoring our inner ache, numbing ourselves with Netflix, perfecting ourselves to the point of exhaustion, all the while out of touch with ourselves, alone in our suffering. We can go on for years emotionally and spiritually malnourished, out of tune with the ancient song of worth, belonging, and purpose being sung over us. As one pastor said four centuries ago, "There are some men and women that have lived forty or fifty years in the world, and have scarce had one hour's discourse with their own hearts all that while."[12]

"Our own depths frighten us!" Ronald Rolheiser writes. "And so we stall, distract ourselves, drug the pain, party and travel, stay busy, try this and that, cling to people and moments, junk up the surface of our lives, and find any and every excuse to avoid being alone and having to face ourselves. We are too frightened to travel inward. But we pay a price for that, a high one: superficiality and shallowness. So long as we avoid the painful journey inward, to the depths of our caverns, we live at the surface."[13]

We know today that the numbing distraction that Rolheiser names is pervasive, but we've normalized it. We seldom wonder what more might be rumbling within our subterranean layers. We relegate our more painful emotions and experiences to the shadows. But, as we've seen, Rebekah's avoidance of her inner ache along with Johanna and Jeff's avoidance of grief disconnected them from vital parts of themselves. After being fired, I spent years working tirelessly to never, ever have to relive the shame and pain, which left me suffering alone, profoundly disconnected. And I'll be honest, the process of coming home to myself was painful. How do you return to a self you really don't like?

Physician and trauma expert Gabor Maté asks, "Why do we get disconnected? Because it is too painful to be ourselves."[14] And when you choose to turn from what happened to you to what's happening within you, it's likely you'll experience some inner resistance. You've been living disconnected for a reason. You were not born separated from yourself, and it's not your native state of living and thriving. That's why it's going to be important to explore how and why you've become disconnected. And it's going to be vital that we chart a course toward home, where reconnection, reunion, and restoration are possible.

Sandhill cranes, monarch butterflies, sea turtles, and many more of God's wondrous creatures have a homing instinct. And so do you. Coming home to yourself—"homing" for short—is a part of the divine design. It's probably why so many of our favorite stories in Scripture are homecoming stories.

God loves to celebrate a return. The Prodigal Son was stuck in his own self-contempt, too, feeling like he was "no longer worthy to be called . . . son" (Luke 15:19), prepared to ask his father for a servant's role. But just as God went out to Adam and Eve, so the father runs to his lost son to celebrate his return:

> While he was still a long way off, his father saw him
> and was filled with compassion for him; he ran to his
> son, threw his arms around him and kissed him.
>
> LUKE 15:20

And so God runs to you, to show you compassion, to offer you the ring, the robe, the sandals, and the feast, all reminders of your irrevocable, image-bearing inheritance. All reminders of your deep worth, belonging, and purpose. All beckoning you home. Can you imagine it?

Would you open yourself to the possibility that God longs

to meet you in whatever experience of disconnection you know? That God longs to celebrate your return? That God longs to call you to a life of freedom and flourishing? If so, there's a journey ahead waiting for you.

RESOURCES

Throughout the book, recommended books are offered as trusted wells of wisdom from which you can draw even deeper resources for your ongoing journey.

- Alison Cook, *The Best of You: Break Free from Painful Patterns, Mend Your Past, and Discover Your True Self in God*
- Martin Laird, *Into the Silent Land: A Guide to the Christian Practice of Contemplation*
- Henri Nouwen, *The Inner Voice of Love: A Journey through Anguish to Freedom*
- Howard Thurman, *The Inward Journey*

Reflection

Throughout the book, these reflections are offered as something you can do on your own, with a friend, or within a small circle of trusted companions.

1. Is there a particular story in this chapter that resonated with you? A sentence (or two) that describes your current experience? If so, write it down and/or share it with someone you trust. Spend some time reflecting on what

stood out to you and what invitation you might sense emerging from this recognition.

2. Did you sense any inner resistance to anything you read? If so, can you track it to a particular thought or theme? Is this something that you can sit with, pay attention to, even share with someone else?

3. We all experience some form of disconnection. What is one unique characteristic of disconnection in your life? And how might you articulate your desire for reconnection and flourishing? What would that look like? What would your inner experience be like? How would your relationships look different after reconnection?

4. How does it feel to consider your God-created worth, belonging, and purpose as evidence of your image-bearing inheritance? What is your inner experience of each of these? What do you need to be reminded of most?

Practice: Come Home to Yourself

Throughout the book, these practices will build upon one another, at times with some overlap and expansion so that you can better experience a growing healing and wholeness.

Intentional breathing

When we're disconnected, we're not grounded—in our breath, in our bodies. Ancient Christians understood this embodied reality and believed the breath to be an access point to God, a place of reconnection. God breathed life into us in Eden (Genesis 2:7), and when the storms of life overwhelm us and the fog devours us, our breathing often becomes shallow. We lose our connection to home. We may even hold our breath. So when we find our way back to our breath, that can also help us find our way back to ourselves, even to God. When you're ready, take some time to breathe in order to reconnect with yourself, with your body, and with God.

It can be helpful to find a quiet space where you can sit down with your feet flat on the floor and your back straight. Take a long, deep breath—in through your nose—then hold it for a few seconds before exhaling slowly through your mouth (as if you're fogging a mirror in front of you, even exhaling audibly with a *haaahhhhhhh*). At the end of your exhale, pause before beginning again. Try this for five to ten minutes at first.

Connecting a prayer to your breathing

There are a variety of prayers you can connect to your breathing exercise as you experience both greater grounding and a return to yourself. I will share two below.

The first is from Psalm 46:10. See if you can't hear the whisper of God's "Where are you?" as you return and reconnect:

> Be still (*in-breath*)
> and know (*out-breath*)
> that I (*in-breath*)
> am God (*out-breath*)

The second is a prayer of St. Patrick dating back to AD 433. This adaptation is a favorite for me because it offers both a spiritual and physical sense of God's presence to you, around you, and within you:

Christ with me (*in-breath*)
Christ before me (*out-breath*)
Christ behind me (*in-breath*)
Christ in me (*out-breath*)
Christ beneath me (*in-breath*)
Christ above me (*out-breath*)
Christ on my right (*in-breath*)
Christ on my left (*out-breath*)
Christ when I lie down (*in-breath*)
Christ when I sit down (*out-breath*)
Christ when I arise (*in-breath*)
Christ in everyone I meet (*out-breath*)

SUFFERING ALONE

How Loneliness Grows a Wound

*Trauma is not what happens to us, but what we hold inside
in the absence of an empathetic witness.*

GABOR MATÉ

PIERCE SITS ACROSS FROM ME on the edge of the couch, his foot anxiously tapping, his eyes scanning my office. I'm his pastor, and he's come to ask for advice about his brother.

Chase, his twin, is a thirtysomething marijuana and opioid user who also attends the church, but who often arrives disheveled and, at times, high. He struggles to keep jobs, sometimes teetering on the edge of homelessness.

Pierce, on the other hand, shows up at church early each Sunday, a bright and charming full participant who seems to be adored by everyone. He dresses well and always appears cheerful.

I don't know either man well, so Pierce tells me a bit of their backstory. They grew up in a wealthy community in the South Bay, their father a high-powered lawyer for top Silicon Valley tech companies. "Dad's affairs and Mom's depression wrecked Chase," Pierce tells me. "It's sad to see him suffer while I've managed to navigate it all so well."

Pierce's comment provokes curiosity, so I ask him about successfully managing these challenges. "Be strong," he says. "People will let you down, but you can always count on yourself!" For Pierce, to be a real man is to never ever need someone. This is the lesson he learned from his father.

As I spend time with Pierce, the fuller picture begins to develop. While Chase's substance use seemed to sabotage any forward progress in career or relationships, Pierce took a different route. He followed his father into law, his new wealth funding an extravagant lifestyle. That included consensual hookups, Pierce admitted. Early on, one son began coping with substances while the other chased success and sex.

But each was running from a painful wound.

Pierce doesn't expect what I share next. "Somewhere along the way, you both lost track of yourselves," I say. I tell him how sad I feel. And he sees and feels my sadness. "You seem so very lonely, too," I tell Pierce, my eyes now welling with tears.

I expect him to evade or disengage, but instead he locks eyes and lets me see him, even the emptiness behind his eyes. "I've been so worried about Chase," he says, "but I sometimes feel as lost as he is." Hanging his head, he finally lets the tears come. And he allows me to sit with him, no longer alone in his pain.

All the Lonely People

Instead of catching the bus after leaving the office that day, I walk down Van Ness Avenue to Market Street, through San Francisco's Castro district and uphill toward our new apartment in Noe Valley, where we moved in hope of a bit less fog. Inspired by Pierce's vulnerability, I walk deliberately, making eye contact when I can with people I don't know.

God's first question, "Where are you?" grows as a longing within me, for myself and for each image bearer designed for worth, belonging, and purpose whom I pass that day.

Unlike my normal routine of walking with eyes averted and ears covered by headphones, I try to stay present amidst a sea of lonely strangers, each with their own story, all in a rush to get somewhere, perhaps even to evade themselves. Continuing on, I find myself pondering the Communion table, where I'd met Chase and Pierce time and again. Do they know how hungry and thirsty they are? Is there any deep satisfaction in the food and drink God offers? In their lostness, do they feel found by God each week? Suddenly, I am overcome with the collective ache of the hundreds of people who come to the table each Sunday with their own stories, their unique pain, and their irrevocable inheritance of worth, belonging, and purpose. Can they let their hearts be touched? I imagine myself asking each one of them the same question: "Where are you?"

Even as I ponder it, I recognize how ironic it is that I, their pastor, feel so lost and lonely too. The truth is, so many of us are alone in our pain and alienated from our deepest selves in God.

"Disconnection in all its guises—*alienation, loneliness, loss of meaning, and dislocation*—is becoming our culture's most plentiful product," addiction and trauma expert Gabor Maté observes. "No wonder we are more addicted, chronically ill, and mentally disordered than ever before, enfeebled as we are by such malnourishment of mind, body, and soul."[1] We're literally lost without connection. We'll go searching, to be sure, just as Pierce and Chase did, surviving off the breadcrumbs of pseudo connection. But it's a recipe for painful isolation, even unhealth.

Yet it's the recognition of this aloneness that is a necessary first step toward reconnection with ourselves, with God, and with those we love.

Alone in our Pain

"To suffer is as human as to breathe," the wise Hogwarts head-master Albus Dumbledore declares.[2] Indeed, none of us are spared from the struggles and sufferings of life within the 1,185 chapters between creation and re-creation. What wounds the soul to its depths, however, is solitary suffering. Here, our pain simmers unaddressed. Here, we begin to forget who we are. And this was the case for Pierce, for me, for each of the people you've been introduced to in the book thus far. The fig-leaved array we've created to protect ourselves from our fear, shame, anger, and more keeps us from being seen and known. God whispers, "Where are you?" but we are lost, even to ourselves. Lost—and alone.

It wasn't meant to be this way, of course. "It is not good for the man to be alone," God says (Genesis 2:18). God's imagination is for a world where humans are offered the chance of real spiritual, emotional, and physical companionship with one another. And in the very first chapter of Scripture, this design is described as *tov meod* in the Hebrew—"very good" (Genesis 1:31).[3] Even before birth, we were designed for connection, for slow growth within a human womb, nine months in complete union with our mothers, literally connected to them for support. This is our very first embodied taste of Eden, of home. And when we're ready, we're born into the world with indispensable, relationship-rich needs to feel safe, seen, soothed, and secure.[4] Connection is the most important need of any infant, essential not just to survival but to human flourishing. Without connection, an infant will die. Indeed, without connection, we cannot truly live.[5] Connection is how we are equipped to navigate life's inevitable trials, how we can experience emotional regulation after we're hurt, how we gain the resilience we need for whatever comes next. Connection is our relational home and the biggest hint of our spiritual inheritance.

But suffering is inevitable. And *suffering alone* is what leaves an incalculable wound. Trauma's best-kept secret, well-articulated by therapist Bonnie Badenoch, is that the "essence of trauma isn't events, but aloneness within them."[6] What has been called a "loneliness epidemic" is now known to be dangerous to both our physical and emotional health. "Being lonely, like other forms of stress, increases the risk of emotional disorders like depression, anxiety and substance abuse," observes John

Leland. "Less obviously, it also puts people at greater risk of physical ailments that seem unrelated, like heart disease, cancer, stroke, hypertension, dementia and premature death."[7] Chronic disconnection magnifies the risks of illness and death, mimicking the impact of smoking fifteen cigarettes a day.[8] Humans literally wither without connection.

Think of it like the thirst your plants experience when they're not sunned and watered. Not long ago, my family and I returned home from vacation to bone-dry plants, their leaves curling and wrinkling. The deep greens had faded, and the plants appeared lifeless—until Sara fed them the water they'd been craving. And so it goes for us in the drought of connection. When we're alone and go it on our own, we, too, begin to wither and fade. In time, we may actually habituate to our dulled and lifeless state, creating the conditions for the festering wound of trauma.

Connection is water and light to weary and withered souls.

In our suffering, we need an empathetic witness, someone to say, "Where are you?," someone who'll see us as we are, someone who'll be with us in it. Absent this, the wound festers, it severs, it tears us up from the inside.

The Slow Wither of Loneliness

Pierce began to see that though he'd never arrive at church without a companion or eat a meal by himself, he was just as lonely as his brother.

And I'd once come to realize that I was withering too. In the first years after I lost my job, I worked hard to assure our family's survival, my survival. Within, I heard the voice of a cruel critic: *You're stuck here, and no one's coming to your rescue. Just tough it out and get through the day.* Little by little, I became like a porcupine, head down, quills out, self-protected. I let no one know how much I was struggling.

But even still, I couldn't shake the growing sense that going it on my own was costing me and those I loved.

An expert on stress and how our bodies hold it, Peter A. Levine writes about how subtle the path to loneliness can be:

> In short, trauma is about loss of connection—to
> ourselves, to our bodies, to our families, to others,
> and to the world around us. This loss of connection is
> often hard to recognize, because it doesn't happen all at
> once. It can happen slowly, over time, and we adapt to
> these subtle changes sometimes without even noticing
> them. These are the hidden effects of trauma, the ones
> most of us keep to ourselves. We may simply sense
> that we do not feel quite right, without ever becoming
> fully aware of what is taking place; that is, the gradual
> undermining of our self-esteem, self-confidence,
> feelings of well-being, and connection to life.[9]

Of course, things happen that throw us out of sorts temporarily. But what Levine is describing is what happens within, a slow habituation to a withered state where it feels like life itself is being drained from us. The stresses of life compound, sending us into a self-protective mode, our body's energies shifting from life-giving connection to life-preserving survival. In time, this withered state we're living in may become our new normal.

This is trauma. And more of us live here than we're willing to admit.

Stressful things happen, to be sure, but stress can grow and metastasize, turning a temporary state of panic into a continuous state of overwhelm. Consider the science of stress for a moment. Therapist Aundi Kolber writes, "A traumatic event includes anything that overwhelms a person's nervous system and ability to cope."[10] In these crucial moments, Kolber notes that our bodies engage in automatic processes within, geared to our survival amidst the overwhelm. No one is exempt; no one is immune. If you're reading this and happen to be human, you've got a nervous system, and that nervous system goes haywire when your survival is threatened in any way. Hormones such as cortisol, adrenaline, and norepinephrine fire within your brain as your heart rate increases and your fight-or-flight response is activated. Your brain's control tower—the prefrontal cortex—goes offline. Other nonessential systems shut down, and key integrative functions cease. At worst, your brain's hippocampus can't do its job of narrating what happened in conscious memory, sabotaging your capacity to remember and process the pain.[11]

Of course, stress doesn't always turn into trauma. Levine notes that "all traumatic events are stressful, but not all stressful events are traumatic."[12] In other words, people may go through identical incidents, but what happens within them may be vastly different. Two people may live through the devastation of a hurricane that destroys their homes and community. One person may find refuge with good friends, allowing her tears to flow freely amidst the empathetic witness of beloved companions who acknowledge her terror and loss. She may come away rattled but not traumatized. The nervous system that jumped in to protect the woman during the hurricane helps her come home to herself when the stress is over. Yet another person may hunker down alone in a hotel, numbing himself amidst the growing rage within. Rather than processing the stress, he may do everything he can to escape it, compounding the overwhelm. One person experiences connection while the other suffers alone.

And this is where I found myself, along with Rebekah, Pierce, Chase, even Jeff and Johanna. None of us could have told you how the shift from connection to survival happened, but it did. In time, we didn't feel like ourselves. Coping became the norm. We didn't notice that our leaves were curling, that our color was fading. We certainly didn't think it was trauma.

Too often, we adapt to states of survival, of coping, of disconnection. It doesn't happen all at once but slowly. In time, we realize we're far from home, internally. This adapted state becomes our new normal, but it's a far cry from the flourishing we were created for.

It is not good for you and me to be alone. Toughing it out is not a virtue. In fact, it's a recipe for overwhelm, exhaustion, isolation, and addiction. God's design for interdependence, relationship, and a vulnerable "knowing and being known" is where we thrive. We need to be seen and known amidst our challenges.

Say "Ouch"

One summer, I convened a support group for survivors of significant spiritual abuse, all of whom were former members of a large church. The stories of harm from this diverse array of folks were held in a space of compassion and curiosity. There were beautiful moments of vulnerability, but there was also a cautiousness that I couldn't quite make sense of.

After some gentle prodding, someone said, "I know it's bad, but she had it a lot worse than I did."

An offhand comment, but with that, the comparison game began. A few more began to minimize their own experiences, gaslighting themselves: "I don't know why I'm crying. . . . I only worked there for five years when some of you worked there so much longer." Instead of witnessing the impact of trauma within them, they began playing a game of "who had it worse."

Somewhere along the way, we learned that there's always someone else, somewhere in the world, who has it worse than we do. And somehow, we've translated this into *stop complaining, it's not that bad.*

"You know, each of you has a nervous system," I told the participants. "And your nervous system isn't comparing what happened. It's coping with the consequences, and it's craving connection." Each of them had suffered, and though their stories were different, their weary and wounded nervous systems needed tender care.

We heal when we attend to what happens within, when we see that each of us is wounded in our own way, each of us coping, each of us often more alone in our pain than we'd dare admit. No matter the supposed size or scope of what happened, we all need care and presence, safety and attunement.

Connection shifts our body out of survival mode and into a state of calm and connectedness again. Psychologist Peter A. Levine, author of *Healing Trauma*, shares a remarkable story of the power of connection amidst acute trauma after he was hit by a car a few years back. The first person on the scene was an off-duty paramedic who attempted to stabilize him, but whose reactive presence and rapid-fire questions were agitating to Peter. His initial pulse reading was 170 bpm. Peter was succumbing to shock. And he felt all alone.

Soon after, a woman came to help, a pediatrician who immediately attended to him as a person. He shares what happened next:

"Please, sit by me." And she did and she grasped my hand. And I could feel her hand and I could smell the scent of her perfume, and the soothingness of her voice. And all of that gave me the feeling that, "I'm not alone," and by having that feeling, I was able to go into my body, into my body, and feel where the shock was locked in my body.[13]

Levine credits her presence and care for his capacity to navigate his body's automatic responses. In fact, shortly after she first attended to him, his pulse dropped to near normal levels, a sign that his body was experiencing safety, regulating itself because another person had met him in his suffering.

What Levine's story tells me is that no matter how we've suffered, we need attuned care and compassion amidst it. We need someone to say "Ouch!" We need a present person who will be with us and who won't minimize what we're feeling. Think of how a good parent responds to a child whether she scrapes her knee or falls out of a tree. A good parent shows up either way, with empathy. A good parent says "Ouch!" no matter the size of the injury. A good parent connects.

And this might begin for you right here as you're reading, as you decide that what you're experiencing—no matter how big or small you perceive it to be—is significant. When you're withering, this kind of reconnection begins to heal you.

"Where are you?" God asks, a kind move toward you amidst your self-protective, porcupine-like posture. God doesn't want you to be alone in your suffering. Don't let the serpent's lies lull you into believing that someone has it worse, or that God has more important things to tend to than to meet you tenderly in your pain. Don't let the serpent convince you to go it on your own, into a land where wandering and withering are inevitable. With a kind "Where are you?" God is addressing *you*. What is the particular pain you carry? How have you carried it on your own? How has it cut you off from vital connection to yourself, to others, to God? What is your experience of it within you?

And what might be possible if you were to let yourself be fully known in it?

The Practice of Befriending Suffering

"Embrace your grief, for there your soul will grow" noted the great twentieth-century psychologist Carl Jung.[14] In chapter 1, I offered the practice of coming home to yourself. Now, I suggest a second practice to build upon it: the practice of befriending your suffering.

In inviting you to befriend suffering, I'm not imagining some masochistic exercise. The *need* to suffer in masochism is yet another means of avoiding or managing real pain. No, I'm more interested in following the invitation of Jesus when he says, "Blessed are those who mourn, for they will be comforted" (Matthew 5:4).

To mourn is to bring your suffering into the light before God and others. To mourn is to refuse to suffer alone anymore. To mourn is to live in truth, to acknowledge that you're hurting, to seek care rather than self-soothing. As Jesus says, "Come to me, all you who are weary and burdened, and I will give you rest" (Matthew 11:28). Indeed, God's credibility for meeting us here is that he suffered in the flesh, experiencing the ache of disconnection and feeling forsaken (Matthew 27:46). Jesus *felt* alone in his suffering. And he cried out. Perhaps we can too.

God runs to you, even in your suffering, longing to reconnect with you. Will you allow yourself to receive God's compassionate care? Will you allow God to see and to know not only what happened to you, but what's happening within you as well? To be sure, many voices will echo the serpent, telling you to go it on your own. But you weren't created to cope alone. And the flourishing you're longing for emerges only as you're known.

While it may sound complicated, I'll often tell people that this practice might just begin with a simple, "Ouch, that hurt!" Yes, it does. That thing that happened to you hurt you. What happens within as a result wounded you. Living life in these 1,185 chapters in between is sometimes painful. It's time to name what hurts, and to name it specifically. Some will tell you that this is a morbid or joyless way of living, but ignoring your pain only leads to further weariness and woundedness. There is no real power in the so-called power of positive thinking because it's a recipe for bypassing your pain, a self-help setup for further hurt. Befriending suffering opens the way for reconnection and joy.

"Suffering is inevitable," South African archbishop Desmond Tutu once noted, "but how we respond to that suffering is our choice. . . . We are fragile creatures, and it is from this weakness, not despite it, that we discover the possibility of true joy."[15] This fragility isn't simply the result of some bad thing we did. It's the reality of being human, limited, even mortal, as theologian Kelly Kapic writes.[16] It is the invitation to acknowledge our weakness, even our neediness. To acknowledge that real strength, even joy, emerges through the embrace of our weakness (2 Corinthians 12:9).

In his lovely work on grief called *The Wild Edge of Sorrow*, therapist Francis Weller muses on the practice of befriending suffering with compassion. He warns us that when we refuse to befriend our suffering, "we will find ourselves acting out of compulsion, reacting to scenes in our life with the same consciousness that was traumatized in the first place." This is where I found myself in my second pastoral role in San Francisco, thousands of miles from where I'd been fired but in the very same body and with the very same consciousness that had experienced that acute pain.

However, when we come home to ourselves, centered and secure, we can approach the pain within us and the suffering outside of us well and wisely, with an empathetic presence. Weller continues, "What we can do is work to maintain our adult presence, keeping it anchored and firmly rooted. This enables us to meet our life with compassion and to receive our suffering without judgments. This is a core piece in our apprenticeship with sorrow."[17]

This isn't to say that we should overidentify with our pain. Too often we say, "I'm depressed" or "I'm addicted" when in reality, we're *feeling* sad or *struggling with* addiction. This distinction makes all the difference.

Your depression, your anxiety, even your addiction, is not core to who you are. Instead, each of these realities within you needs the balm of reconnection, needs a witness to its pain. You bear God's image, and you are "hidden with Christ in God" (Colossians 3:3) and "rooted and grounded in love" (Ephesians 3:17, ESV). Anchored here at home within, you can notice your pain within not *as you*, but as a *part* of you, perhaps an *experience* you're having or a way you're currently *coping*. Anchored here at home within, you can join the Spirit of God within you as an empathetic witness to your own pain, a vital part of the healing process.

There is an old hymn that offers you an invitation:

Come, ye disconsolate, where'er ye languish;
Come to the mercy-seat, fervently kneel;
Here bring your wounded hearts, here tell your anguish,
Earth has no sorrow that heaven cannot heal.[18]

You don't have to suffer alone. Bring it into the light and let your leaves unfurl.

RESOURCES

- Amanda Held Opelt, *A Hole in the World: Finding Hope in Rituals of Grief and Healing*
- Dennae Pierre, *Healing Prayers and Meditations to Resist a Violent World*
- Curt Thompson, *The Soul of Shame: Retelling the Stories We Believe about Ourselves*
- Francis Weller, *The Wild Edge of Sorrow: Rituals of Renewal and the Sacred Work of Grief*

Reflection

Even if we experienced great care growing up, almost everyone has some story of suffering alone at some point. And almost everyone can think of some message they learned about being tough or strong or independent.

1. Can you think of an experience from any period of your life when you suffered alone? What was it? How did it feel? If you were eventually met in it, how did that help? If you weren't, how does it feel even today reflecting on what it was like to suffer alone?

2. How did your family talk about painful things? How were you attended to when you were hurt? Was there a particular mantra that was spoken or an implied expectation about how to get over it or through it quickly? See if you can name some of the childhood lessons you learned about how you were supposed to deal with pain.

3. Has suffering alone become normalized for you, perhaps to the point that no one really knows what you're experiencing? If so, how might it feel to open yourself up to God by acknowledging that it hurts? How would it feel to share some of what you're feeling with a friend?

4. We sometimes tend to minimize our suffering through comparison. How have you done this? What is it like to consider that your unique struggle—no matter what it is— is the very place where God meets you?

Practice: Befriend Your Suffering

In coming home to yourself, you learned to reconnect, to breathe and to ground, and to attend to God's kind "Where are you?" Now, in this practice, you'll learn to begin to name the ache within.

Writing your laments

Psalms of lament were spoken as an antidote to suffering alone. They were pleas to God in the midst of isolating pain. It can be helpful to write your own reflection in the spirit of these biblical psalms. There are psalms of individual lament—Psalm 3, 5-7, 13, 17, 22, 25-28, 32, 38, 39, 42, 43, 51, 54-57, 59, 61, 63, 64, 69-71, 86, 88, 102, 109, 120, 130, and 140-43. There are also psalms of communal lament—Psalm 44, 74, 79, 80, 83, and 89.[19] You can begin by reading through some of these to see which one uses language or a tone that resonates with your own soul or struggle. You might then just grab a pen and a journal and begin writing your own prayer of lament. Capture on paper what feels faithful to your experience without trying to mimic the psalmist too closely, recognizing that God wants to hear your unique experience. As you listen to God's "Where are you?" perhaps you can honestly name what you are experiencing.

Separating and attending

Amidst disconnection, you can slowly begin to believe that you are your emotions, or even your addictions. Sometimes you may be so overwhelmed by an emotion or an experience that you can't return to yourself in order to approach your pain from a place of care and compassion. In these moments, it can be helpful simply to name what's happening within. This exercise can help you both return to yourself and begin to befriend and name how you're suffering. Practice the following exercise:

- *I am not my _____ [sadness, rage, panic, shame, etc.]. I am simply feeling _____ [sadness, rage, panic, shame, etc.]. This isn't me. It's a part of me that needs my care and compassion. At my core, I'm loved by God and created for worth, belonging, and purpose.*

or

- *I am not my _____ [addictive tendency]. I am simply coping right now by _____ [name the way you're coping]. This isn't who I am; it's just the way I am dealing with my pain right now. At my core, I'm loved by God and created for worth, belonging, and purpose.*

In this practice, you might see if you're able to identify where you are feeling particular feelings or sensations in your body. Then place your hand there (over your chest, on your cheeks, or on your belly, for example), and breathe in slowly, according to the exercise in chapter 1 (see pages 29–30). On the out-breath, imagine yourself breathing compassion into this area of your body or into this particular internal feeling or sensation.

Companionship

Practice asking for care. Practice being known. When we struggle alone, we're more prone to becoming overwhelmed, even traumatized. Is there someone you can invite into this reading and reflection with you? Perhaps someone you can find a one-hour slot each week to process with? Maybe even someone you can engage the "separating and attending" exercise with? If so, begin practicing a kind of soul companionship where you can know and be known. Simply start with the question "Where are you?" and see where it leads. Maybe the examples in this chapter offer some helpful connections to your own life and show how each of us, like Adam and Eve, wander and get lost. Be as honest as you're able. And then follow this up with another question: "Is this where I want to be?" Or "What do I long for?" Begin here, and we'll build on this in the pages to come.

THE BODY TELLS A STORY

Learning to Listen

I have calmed and quieted my soul, like a weaned child with its mother; my soul within me is like a weaned child.

PSALM 131:2,
ADAPTED FROM THE ESV AND NRSV

ERIN IS A BUSY MOM IN HER MID-THIRTIES, not given to slowing down. After all, she has three children to raise and a husband whose business travel leaves her parenting solo quite often. During one of our first sessions together, I ask her how she is doing. She blushes and blurts out, "I'm running on empty, and I didn't even see the warning light."

Erin has learned to ignore her gut feelings, unaware of the storm brewing within. She has become more and more impatient with her youngest, sometimes ignoring his cries altogether. She has lost weight at a pace that has worried her closest friends. They notice her increasing distance—not answering texts, not showing up for coffee at their weekly gathering. She can't sleep at night. She sometimes skips her scheduled therapy sessions. And she doesn't really feel like eating. After accidentally falling asleep and missing her children's afternoon school pickup, she calls me in a panic, apologizing profusely for missing some sessions and asking for my earliest appointment.

During our next session, Erin expects a guilt-laden chastisement, perhaps some condemnation for being a bad client and a bad parent. But I sense her quiet suffering and meet her with a tender gaze, thanking her for asking for what she needed. She sits on my couch and exhales, tears immediately welling. "That feels strange and good," she says with a delighted smile. Her body seems to unfurl, her hands releasing their grasp on the arms of my office chair.

"I think your body is happy you're back," I tell her.

"Yeah, I've been kind of pushing everything down, kind of ignoring it all," she says.

"There's no rush, but maybe you can begin to pay attention a bit more to what's happening within you," I note.

She closes her eyes and places her hand on her chest, rubbing it gently, tears again emerging. "It's time," she says.

Our Inner Dashboard

Sometimes we drive inattentive to the dashboard warning lights flashing before our eyes. Our lives are busy. There are emails to return, groceries to buy, meetings to attend, bills to pay, leaky faucets to fix, diapers to change, bosses to please, and snow-covered driveways to shovel—at least in West Michigan. Our bodies adjust to the adrenaline-fueled survival game of life. We keep our heads above water most of the time, our ailing and weary bodies drifting below, tossed in the currents. We ignore what's happening within.

The kinds of symptoms that emerge when we ignore our warning lights may seem subtle at first. Imagine an inner dashboard that might alert you when signs of stress become noteworthy. Most of us can manage a few yellow warning lights, or so we think. *I can handle it!* we tell ourselves. But sprinkle in a few red warning lights and things get messier. I know someone who'd cover any vehicle warning light that came on with black electrical tape so as to avoid the hassle of car repairs. That is, until he found himself unable to brake one day, leading to a collision with a large truck.

Indeed, when we don't have the words, our bodies inevitably tell the story of where we really are. Sometimes, our bodies will even do drastic things to get our attention. This is what happened to me. After several years in San Francisco, my workaholism caught up with me. I thought hard work and success might dim the churning anxiety within, but they just covered the warning lights. And then it happened—all the lights came on at once while I was on a dream vacation in Cabo, Mexico. The pain in my stomach became severe, joined by lower back pain and a growing fever. With each passing day, I'd medicate with more ibuprofen. I woke one night in such pain that I stood in a hot shower as long as I could, letting the pulsing water fall on my throbbing lower back. My wife and friends finally convinced me to go to a local hospital.

If we refuse to say "Help!" and if we're unable to cry out "Ouch, that hurts," our bodies may speak for us. And my body had an important story it wanted me to know.

The capable doctors ran multiple tests before an ultrasound revealed the culprit—gallstones. What should have been a fairly normal gallbladder removal was complicated by sepsis, my system having turned toxic. My defiance of suffering had only caused more suffering, and my body told the story. I was sick and hurting. Truth is, I'd been sick and hurting for some time.

Though I'd been in therapy and was continuing to heal in that space, I discovered the depth of my disconnection in the weeks after my gallbladder surgery, as I reflected on how my body had absorbed years of stress. An unfortunate consequence of this disconnection is that we "often become expert at ignoring . . . gut feelings," prone to "numbing awareness of what is played out inside," as Bessel van der Kolk, author of *The Body Keeps the Score*, notes.[1] I realized that though I'd told stories of what had happened to me in therapy, I'd ignored how my body held these stories—what was happening within me. I saw that I'd disregarded multiple warning lights over the years—exhaustion, IBS symptoms, sleeplessness, shame, hypervigilance, panic, dread.

"Where are you?" God asked me. And I sensed then that I needed to pay attention much more carefully than I'd thought.

Learning the Warning Signs

If it's helpful, consider your own internal dashboard for a moment. Imagine a place for your thoughts, your emotions, your bodily sensations, your relational energy, and your behavior, all of which may go unnoticed if you don't bring intentional awareness to your body.[2] In the image below you'll see some examples of each of these. You might take just a moment to write down which words resonate with your own experience. You can note which give you a sense of pause or caution (a yellow warning light to slow down and pay attention) and which give you a sense of more significant alarm (a red warning light to stop and attend right now).

Thoughts: all-or-nothing thinking, confusion, delusions, inattentiveness, indecision, judgment of self or others, memory problems, obsessiveness, self contempt, self-doubt, suicidal ideation, trouble concentrating or orienting in time

Relational energy: angry outbursts, avoiding particular places, avoiding people to preserve energy, constant checking up on others, constant scanning, relying on others to meet your needs

SYMPTOMS

Emotions: anger, desperation, distrust, emptiness, fear, guilt, hopelessness, irritation, listlessness, loneliness, numbness, overwhelm, panic, rage, resentment, shame, sadness

Behavior: addictive behaviors, busyness without boundaries, job losses, lack of self-care, not getting out of bed, overeating or overdrinking, self-harm

Body: aches, blurred vision, chronic pain, disconnection, exhaustion, headaches, heartburn, hypervigilance, irritable bowel syndrome, nausea, out-of-body feelings, racing heart, sleeplessness

In the case of my client, Erin, we worked to create her own list of where she was experiencing yellow and red warning lights on her internal dashboard:

YELLOW	RED
Sadness	Emptiness
IBS	Fear
Withdrawal	Desperation
Heartburn	Self-judgment
Irritation	Sleeplessness
Shame	Exhaustion
Angry outbursts	Lack of self-care

Erin was stunned as she stood back and looked at her list. "I can't believe I'm still standing," she said.

The practice of paying attention, as Erin did in this exercise, is important on a scientific level as well. The warning lights on your personal dashboard are symptoms of stress that can become wounds of trauma if neglected, disconnecting you in ways that hurt yourself and others. They are the first sign that allow you, and perhaps a trusted friend or counselor, to know what more might be happening within you. And with careful attunement and attention to your inner experience, you can become curious about what these signals are telling you. In this way, you begin to provide a concrete answer to the question, "Where are you?" What has been ignored is now on paper, a clear invitation to pay attention and begin to heal what's within.

It helps me to know that Scripture offers many pictures of this. King David himself listened to his body and offered its groanings in prayer before God:

> My wounds fester and are loathsome
>   because of my sinful folly.
> I am bowed down and brought very low;
>   all day long I go about mourning.
> My back is filled with searing pain;
>   there is no health in my body.
> I am feeble and utterly crushed;
>   I groan in anguish of heart.
>
> All my longings lie open before you, Lord;
>   my sighing is not hidden from you.
> My heart pounds, my strength fails me;
>   even the light has gone from my eyes.
> My friends and companions avoid me because of my
>   wounds;
>   my neighbors stay far away.
> PSALM 38:5-11

David's attunement to his pounding heart, his searing pain, his unhealth, even his anguish—both here and in many other psalms—opens the possibility for you to attune and attend to your pain too. David's prayer paints the picture of a man desperate, eager to come out of hiding and to be known by God in his suffering. This is your invitation too. The call to pay attention isn't an invention of a modern therapist, but a call to faithful presence—to ourselves, to God, to each other.

Lost in the Storm and Fog

Remember Pierce, the Silicon Valley lawyer from the last chapter who'd followed his father's career path and ways of coping? Successful by all accounts in the world's eyes, Pierce had ignored symptoms of underlying pain for years. He'd learned to navigate life with too little sleep and too much drink, with a constant buzzing anxiety within and a relentless drive to chase after experiences that he thought would fulfill him. In time, these symptoms felt like familiar friends instead of the warning lights they actually were, cues from his body that something was dreadfully wrong. As a result, he wasn't paying attention.

If he had been, Pierce would have seen that he had resided in a place of constant inner tumult for most of his life. Stress trumped security in his early years; his parents were largely emotionally unavailable, taxing his nervous system from his first days. Unlike his twin brother, Pierce gravitated toward his father, idolizing him, even amidst his marital unfaithfulness and exhausting workaholism. When the sense of aloneness or disconnection became too pronounced, he'd self-soothe in ways that filled the empty gap for a moment but only escalated his sense of isolation and pain in the long run. Feeling unseen and longing for connection, he went with his dad on a business trip while still a teenager, only to be drawn into a sexual encounter while away from home. He recalled both the exhilaration and loneliness of it, and in time a repeated pattern of exhilaration and loneliness became normal for him.

Pierce lived in what I call Storm.[3] From a nervous system perspective, Storm is a state of hyperarousal, where our sympathetic system is activated in an effort to survive a perceived threat of any kind. Our blood pressure and heart rate are elevated, adrenaline pumping, with involuntary responses of *fight*, *flight*, *fawn*, or *find*.[4]

In *fight*, we're stuck in "enemy mode,"[5] defending and protecting ourselves, demanding from others, frustrated and resistant. In *flight*, we're anxious and vigilant, avoiding anything that we perceive as threatening. In *fawn*, we're overly appeasing and compliant, escaping the tension of possible conflict. And in *find*, we're desperately searching for someone to soothe and protect us.

These responses are our bodies' attempts to keep us safe and get our immediate needs met, however we can. These states are meant to be temporary—quick fixes to make the warning light stop flashing. The issue is that, for many, this Storm begins to feel like home. We may adapt to life here, staying for years, even for decades, suffering alone.

While some are lost in a Sympathetic Storm, others are stuck in a Fog. Still a means of survival, this is the opposite end of the spectrum, our bodies slogging into a perpetually dulled state where we experience chronic weariness, shame, depression, disengagement, and unhealthy self-soothing. This is a state of hypoarousal. And in contrast to the Storm-like churning of the sympathetic nervous system, this Fog-like state is governed by the parasympathetic nervous system. Psychologist Stephen Porges calls this the dorsal vagal state, which helps us understand how our primitive vagus nerve does what it's been doing for ages in all animals, including fish, in times of danger— shutting us down to protect us.

If in a Sympathetic Storm one is mobilized to actively protect and defend, the Dorsal Fog is a place of immobilization. Here we may *freeze* or *fold*. In *freeze*, we experience a clash between our desire to mobilize and our desire to self-protect.[6] We may feel panicky, rigid, and stuck. Our muscles tense, our eyes widen, and our heart rate speeds up. If the threat passes, we may relax. But if it doesn't, we may *fold*. In *fold*, we experience a chemical bath to numb the pain, leaving us foggy and dissociative. Our heart rate lowers, our muscles relax, and vital connection processes within us shut off, possibly rendering us unable to remember what happened that led us to fold. We may feel ashamed and helpless, becoming severely depressed or submissive to someone harming us or to the overwhelm. At worst, we may completely shut down.

This is where Pierce's brother, Chase, lived the majority of his life. From an early age, Chase recalled feeling more aligned with his mother, even amidst her depression and emotional unavailability. Considered the more sensitive of the brothers, Chase grew to resent his father's busyness and infidelities, and internalized a sense that he wasn't worth his father's time and attention. Feeling powerless to connect to either his father or mother and wrestling with a constant sense of shame, worthlessness, and emptiness, Chase found some comfort during his teenage years when he smoked weed with his friends. As an adult, he'd make enough money to pay for a bed at night and fund whatever substance he required to keep his pain at bay. Numbing dulled his agitated emotions and disconnected him from a sense of his parents' abandonment, leaving him in a perpetual state of foggy dissociation.

Pierce was stuck in the Storm, constantly churning internally. Chase couldn't escape the Fog, a thick blanket that didn't let the light through. Both were far from home. And for each, life in these states had become normal. Their dashboard warning lights had been ignored for years. Anyone who knew them could tell that, though twins, their personalities were markedly different. But what couldn't be explained by personality style was how stuck they both were.

Homing

One of the ways we can better recognize what weather pattern is raging is to feel the warmth of the sun, to know the glorious, clear-weathered view of the horizon. Of home.

I was born on Long Island and went to college in Iowa. Sara and I have lived in Chicago, Orlando, San Francisco, and Holland and Grand Rapids, Michigan. That's a lot of transition! Most recently, we downsized as empty nesters into a small, midcentury modern house. Its clean lines, flat roof, and large windows allow for views of the lovely oak and hickory trees behind it. We fell in love with the house, but the anxiety of the move and the process of unpacking left my body in a state of unrest for at least a couple of months. It took some time, but as I lay in bed one lazy Sunday afternoon watching the last browning leaves of autumn fall, I whispered to myself, "Home."

Perhaps you know the feeling. When a house becomes a home, it's a place where you can relax, where you can be completely yourself, where the cares of the day seem to melt away. If you travel much, you know the disruption of being away from home, especially if you're in hotels or crossing time zones. And if you're in tune with your body, you'll likely long for home again, for your own bed and pillow, and for the fresh-brewed coffee you don't have to pay a small fortune for.

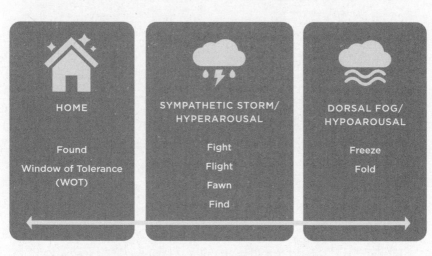

HOME	SYMPATHETIC STORM/ HYPERAROUSAL	DORSAL FOG/ HYPOAROUSAL
Found	Fight	Freeze
Window of Tolerance (WOT)	Flight	Fold
	Fawn	
	Find	

Now imagine a great bay window in your internal Home offering a view of all that is good and beautiful. Psychiatrist Daniel J. Siegel calls this the window of tolerance (WOT), a space within you where you feel present, grounded, and emotionally regulated.[7] He describes this WOT as a place of calm within you where you're able to feel your feelings in a right-sized way and act from a centered place. The safer you feel, the wider the window is and the more able you are to experience all that life throws at you, without being pulled into Storm or Fog. And the good news is that you can cultivate a life in this Home, expanding your window, opening yourself to what Jesus calls life abundant (John 10:10, ESV).

When the writer of Proverbs invites you to "guard your heart, for everything you do flows from it" (Proverbs 4:23), I suspect this is exactly what Porges, Siegel, and other psychological cartographers of the self are referring to. Though they likely don't know it, they are signaling the physiological experience of living from our true selves, anchored in God. Home begins in Eden, its memory still with us. As Frederick Buechner reminds us, "At the innermost heart, at the farthest reach, of our remembering, there is peace. The secret place of the Most High is there. Eden is there, the still waters, the green pastures. Home is there."[8] You might even imagine this place as the warm living room in your very center, right beside that spacious bay window (WOT), a place for you to return to when it feels like the Fog is looming or a Storm is brewing.

Living from our true selves, "hidden with Christ in God" (Colossians 3:3). Living in connection and safety and in our physiological WOT, experiencing the spacious delight of our social engagement system.

HOME

"Rooted and grounded in love" (Ephesians 3:17, ESV). Calm, restful, connected, curious, relaxed, hopeful, open, flexible, aware, joyful; anchored in our sense of worth, belonging, and purpose.

Indeed, Home is within the "still waters" of God's love and care (Psalm 23:2, KJV). It is where we discover God as our refuge, our safe place amid danger (Psalm 46:1). Home is being "hidden with Christ in God" (Colossians 3:3) and "rooted and grounded in love" (Ephesians 3:17, ESV). It is where we're anchored in a sense of our image-bearing worth, belonging, and purpose (Genesis 1:27). And we're not alone here, because the Holy Spirit dwells in us and with us always, even when we've strayed far from Home (1 Corinthians 6:19). As Martin Laird writes, "God is our homeland. And the homing instinct of the human being is homed on God."[9]

When you do stray, as you're apt to do, God awakens your inner homing beacon with the curious and kind question: "Where are you?" And God runs to greet you with joy and compassion upon your return (Luke 15:20). Home is your access point, always fixed. You may drift, but you'll never become completely untethered, because nothing can separate you from God's love (Romans 8:39). Your heart may wander, but your deepest longing is for Home, because it is the only place you'll find shalom, the wholeness and flourishing for which you were created (Psalm 42).

Just as we work to understand our body's warning lights, it's important to learn what it feels like to be at home in your body when you're centered and secure, rested and resilient. St. Teresa of Ávila wrote, "What could be worse than not being at home in our own house? What hope do we have of finding rest outside of ourselves if we cannot be at ease within? . . . If we don't cultivate peace at home, we will not find it in alien places."[10] Cultivating this peace at home is an active process, one that invites each of us to familiarize ourselves with our lived experience of Home.

For me, there is a certain grounding in my body and attentiveness to my senses that makes me feel alive and present. I'm not floating above myself as I'm sometimes apt to do when I feel a bit disconnected or even dissociative, but I'm anchored, as if gravity is pulling me down into myself. I'm breathing deeply, something I don't do when I'm rushing about. I'm relaxed and spacious, an elusive reality when my schedule is packed and I'm racing from meeting to meeting. I have access to all of my emotions, but they don't overwhelm me. I feel connected to myself, to God, to those I love. Mostly, I feel like myself, and I kind of like myself when I'm here, which isn't always the case.

You might just take a moment right now to get curious about your own experience of this spiritual and physiological state of Home. You might even journal as you consider these questions: When do you feel most at Home? Where? With whom? What conditions in your life contribute to this lived sense of being at Home? On the flip side, when do you feel disconnected, alienated, and out of touch with yourself and others?

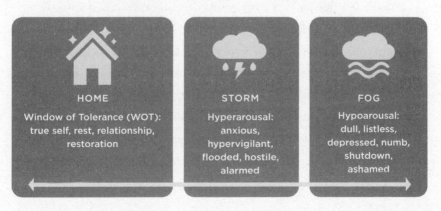

HOME	STORM	FOG
Window of Tolerance (WOT): true self, rest, relationship, restoration	Hyperarousal: anxious, hypervigilant, flooded, hostile, alarmed	Hypoarousal: dull, listless, depressed, numb, shutdown, ashamed

The Practice of Paying Attention

"Search me, God, and know my heart," King David asks in Psalm 139:23. I suspect he knew that God was already looking. Perhaps he read the first chapters of Genesis and heard God asking, "Where are you, David?"

Truth is, we know a lot about David. He leaves very little hidden. Of the 150 psalms, he wrote nearly half, offering us more than a glimpse into his glaring vulnerabilities, his desperate fear, his self-sabotaging ways.[11] In the early centuries of the church, St. Augustine would follow his lead, devoting nine of the thirteen chapters of his autobiographical *Confessions* to his own harrowing story, honestly naming the detours and disorders of a soul in search of Home. And these two men were not the only ones who paid attention.

St. Teresa of Ávila wrote about her own somatic symptoms, likely vestiges of childhood trauma. The English preacher Charles Spurgeon detailed his consuming depression in vulnerable letters to his parishioners, a depression that sometimes kept him from preaching on Sundays.[12] St. Thérèse of Lisieux chronicled her battles with doubt, feeling enveloped in darkness, even abandoned by God. And Thomas Merton's autobiographical work *The Seven Storey Mountain* details his own painful story, naming how his own hurt spilled over, even in a narcissism that harmed others. These women and men paid attention to what was happening within. Their stories compel us, and their lost-and-found journeys give us permission to name the realities of our own wandering and wayward hearts.

Their stories invite us to home in on our own hearts, as the psalmists invite us to do.

The saints and psalmists practiced paying attention, and this was well before therapists began touting the benefits of analysis, introspection, and self-awareness. Perhaps this might bolster your own courage. I sometimes lament the fact that the practice of paying attention isn't immediately thought to be the faithful habit of every growing Christian. Beginning with St. Augustine and throughout Christian tradition, it has been called the practice of self-knowledge, an invitation to honesty whose fruit is humility. So it saddens me that a flannelgraph faith is too often the norm within our churches. Attending to what happens within us isn't merely work reserved for the therapy room. Perhaps it ought to be invited even in worship, as King David modeled.

Today I hear people of faith say, "Don't focus on yourself; focus on others." After writing *When Narcissism Comes to Church*, I heard people mistakenly refer to narcissism as self-focus. Ironically, those who tend toward narcissism are radically out of touch with themselves. They're disconnected— from themselves, from God, from others. They're not attuned and possess no self-knowledge. In fact, the practice of paying attention is actually an antidote to narcissistic disconnection. Homing in on what's happening within opens our hearts to love, to worship, to serve in freedom and with full hearts.

The practice of paying attention builds on the previous two exercises, and may also awaken a need for them. A stay in a Mexican hospital got my attention in a way prior therapy hadn't. And so it goes for some of us. Our bodies tell the story, quite honestly. They may just give us the best data around what's happening within. And we had best begin to listen. Our bodies were designed to flourish. And they'll tell us when we're not.

"If you're willing to pay attention to and dialogue with what's happening inside of you, you'll find that your body already knows the answers about how to live a full, present, connected, and healthy life," says Hillary L. McBride, author of *The Wisdom of Your Body*.[13] And what she means is that our God-created bodies are already equipped to reconnect and be restored with some intentional practice on our end. The poet Mary Oliver echoes this when she writes, "Though Eden is lost its loveliness remains in the heart."[14] Even if you've lived for years mired in symptoms and states that have become normal for you, your body can and will respond as you reengage and reconnect to it.

It can be scary at first. Most of us went years ignoring our gut intuition, our somatic cues, even our hunger, thirst, or need for sleep. Yes, we've become experts at ignoring our bodies and our emotions. In certain Christian spaces, attending to our bodies and emotions is suspect, a sign that perhaps we're following our feelings rather than God. Many of us thought our emotions and bodies were problems to be solved rather than sources of wisdom to be honored, as King David reveals in Psalm 38.

But if David's words teach us anything, they teach us to be honest. They teach us to name what we're feeling. They teach us to listen. There is no mental work-around to heal our wounds, no training manual to memorize, no verse to claim some miraculous victory that sidesteps real, honest engagement with God and with the stories our bodies are telling. The truth is that we can follow our feelings *to* God; we can listen to our bodies in order to long more deeply for God's grace, presence, and healing.

And that's what that first, ancient story in Scripture reveals too. When God approached Adam and Eve with a compassionate "Where are you?" they were already disconnected, mired in anxiety, hidden amidst their own storming hyperarousal within. Searing shame severed them from themselves, even their own bodies. Their quickly-sewn-together fig-leaved garments were a survival strategy for life outside of Eden. But they were not well. Indeed, they were far from Home. Maybe you know the feeling.

Genesis 3 is often told as a story of cosmic tragedy, a proof text for all that went wrong. And, indeed, you need only read the chapters to come to realize the calamity of self-sufficiency, of a life lived in chronic disconnection. But even amidst this, don't miss the stunning reality that God pursues, God attunes, and God blesses, even tending to the bodies of Adam and Eve, highlighted by this compassionate act: "The LORD God made garments of skin for Adam and his wife and clothed them" (Genesis 3:21).

Cole Arthur Riley in *This Here Flesh* highlights this stunning and sometimes overlooked moment:

On the day the world began to die, God became a seamstress. This is the moment in the Bible that I wish we talked about more often. When Eve and Adam eat from the tree, and decay and despair begin to creep in, when they learn to hide from their own bodies, when they learn to hide from each other—no one ever told me the story of a God who kneels and makes clothes out of animal skin for them.

I remember many conversations about the doom and consequence imparted by God after humans ate from that tree. I learned of the curses, too, and could maybe even recite them. But no one ever told me of the tenderness of this moment. . . .

When shame had replaced Eve's and Adam's dignity, God became a seamstress. He took the skin off of his creation to make something that would allow humans to stand in the presence of their maker and one another again.[15]

Even in that ancient story, God compassionately attended to Adam and Eve, to anxious hearts and shame-riddled bodies. God does the same for you.

Perhaps your shame keeps you disconnected from yourself, from your emotions, even your body. Perhaps your wounds keep you either in a constant fight-or-flight cycle or in chronic shutdown. Your body tells a story. Will you listen?

Home, as Mary Oliver hints at, is your deepest memory. Trust that your body will show you the way. Listen to it. Befriend it. Greet every experience as a message from a wandering exile within, longing to be received with compassion upon their return. The same God who attuned so compassionately to Adam and Eve comes in the flesh, embodied, one with us in order to bear our wounds, in order to forgive us, in order to heal us. Like the father who wraps his prodigal son in the family's "best robe" (Luke 15:22), so God the seamstress attends to you with great curiosity, care, and compassion. Perhaps you can let yourself feel it too.

RESOURCES

- Diana Gruver, *Companions in the Darkness: Seven Saints Who Struggled with Depression and Doubt*
- Aundi Kolber, *Try Softer: A Fresh Approach to Move Us out of Anxiety, Stress, and Survival Mode—and into a Life of Connection and Joy*
- Hillary L. McBride, *The Wisdom of Your Body: Finding Healing, Wholeness, and Connection through Embodied Living*
- Tara M. Owens, *Embracing the Body: Finding God in Our Flesh and Bone*
- Cole Arthur Riley, *This Here Flesh: Spirituality, Liberation, and the Stories That Make Us*
- Daniel J. Siegel, *Mindsight: The New Science of Personal Transformation*

Reflection

1. What has been your relationship with your body and your emotions? What lessons did you learn from home or from church about how to navigate both?

2. Take some time to describe what Home feels like in your body today. On your very best days, when you feel calm and connected, when your emotions are rightsized, when you can handle a bit more, what do you experience within you? What are the conditions around you that make this possible?

3. Your dashboard alerts you to symptoms you might have been ignoring for some time. Take a few minutes to write down some symptoms you have encountered in the last several days as you experience them through your thoughts, emotions, bodily sensations, behaviors, and relational energy. Which of these, if any, are a surprise to you? Who might you invite into a conversation about what you're experiencing?

4. As you consider the Storm and the Fog, is there one you've spent more time in? Are there particular seasons of your life where you can see yourself living in that pattern? Do you feel stuck in one or the other right now?

Practice: Pay Attention

Embodied prayer

Read all of Psalm 38. Notice everywhere David describes his thoughts, emotions, bodily experiences/sensations, behaviors, or relationships with others or God. What words or phrases stand out to you? Why? If you have a partner or a small group you're doing this with, compare your reflections on how David describes his experience. Then see if you might be able to craft your own psalm by engaging your thoughts, emotions, body, behaviors, and relational energy.

Reconnecting with your body

A daily or regular *body scan* practice has the benefit of being both immensely relaxing and profoundly helpful for feeling a deeper connection with your body. Some meditation apps lead you through body scans, and you can find other guides online.[16] For some who are particularly disconnected from their bodies, this can help quickly identify areas where there may be tension or discomfort. If more painful memories or sensations are evoked, it will be important to work with a trauma-informed therapist for care. Beyond body scans, engaging in a regular practice of yoga—including trauma-informed yoga—can be deeply healing.[17] Or a simple exercise in mindful walking can awaken you to your body and your surroundings in a new way.[18]

Being with

Hillary L. McBride writes, "If I could sum up all my years of clinical training and research in one statement, it would be this: *We heal when we can be with what we feel.*"[19] Choose one symptom from your list. It might be obsessive thinking, a clenched jaw, or anxiety that you sense in your gut and chest. Anything will do. See if you can sense God's Spirit within you aligning with your own desire to simply "be with" this experience. See if you can bring curiosity, compassion, and care as you stay with whatever you're experiencing and practice breathing according to the exercise in chapter 1 (see pages 29–30). Humans tend to disconnect from difficult emotions, thoughts, and sensations, so this exercise is designed simply to reverse that tendency and retrain your body and brain to attune and attend rather than ignore. As you do this, you may also engage these words:

- *Right now I am choosing not to numb or distract, but simply to be with _____ [my sadness, my headache, my anger, etc.]. In the past, I would _____ [describe how you'd disconnect], but now with God's Spirit in me, I will stay connected and present to whatever comes. I'll receive God's compassion and offer myself compassion.*

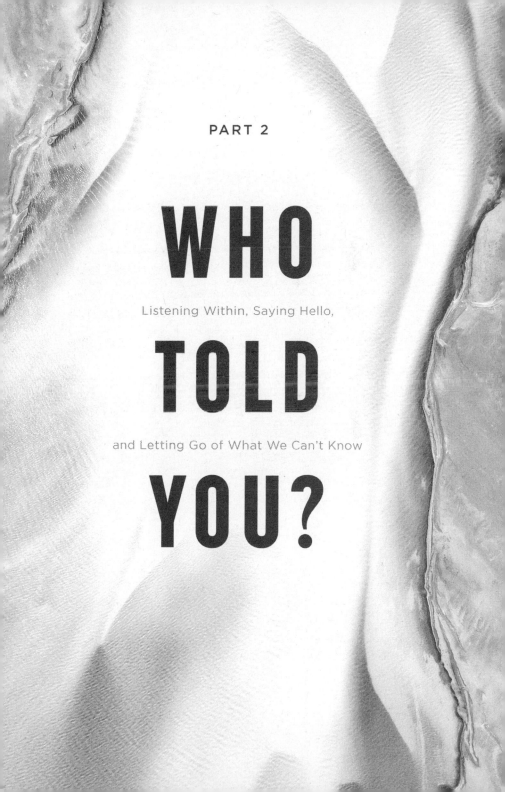

PART 2

WHO

Listening Within, Saying Hello,

TOLD

and Letting Go of What We Can't Know

YOU?

WHOSE VOICES DO WE HEAR?

How Our Earliest Stories Shape Our Souls

*Our first and most important spiritual task is to claim God's
unconditional love for ourselves. To remember who we truly are
in the memory of God. . . . That we are God's beloved.*

HENRI J. M. NOUWEN

THOUGH GOD CREATED A GARDEN in which all of Adam and
Eve's needs would be met, the serpent raised the possibility that
something was missing, that God couldn't be counted on to
take care of them. Shame eroded their sense of worth, alienation
overcame their sense of belonging, disillusionment drowned
out their sense of purpose.

We read the story of Genesis 3 with such rapt attention
because it's our own. We, too, were lulled to sleep in the garden
and lost track of God's original whisper over us. "Who told
you?" God asks. And we look back, retracing our steps. We
wonder whose voice it was who offered us a counternarrative,
a story not worthy of Eden's joy, goodness, and delight. If we

listen carefully, each of us can hear the slithering serpent's gas-lighting lies murmuring within us. These lies undermine our sense of worth, belonging, and purpose—contradicting our image-bearing glory and convincing us that we're not worth it, that God isn't interested in being with us, that we have no future.

While some might contend that our core problem as humans is that we think too highly of ourselves, I'd argue that most of us live with an underlying sense of worthlessness, alienation, and disillusionment. We achieve, trying to prove our worth. We grasp for love. We clamor for meaning. Here we struggle, wounded, weary, and wandering, as the riptide quickly pulls us away from Home, out into the storming seas where we're tossed about once again, mired in the traumatic tumult. I've never known anyone who hasn't wrestled with deep questions of worth, belonging, and purpose. Even those who've been loved deeply and held securely eventually find their way east of Eden, wandering in the wilderness, questioning God's goodness and their "enoughness" in God.

I wish I could awaken every day, freshly reminded that noth-ing can separate me from God's love. But sometimes within minutes of my alarm sounding, I can feel the stirring of restless-ness within, the foreboding sense that there is too much to do and that I'm not up to it all, the lies that God doesn't care and that I'm not enough. The ancient trauma narrated in Genesis 3 still hovers near, a primal wound within that speaks the lie that we're doomed to a life of achieving, chasing, even grasping for the inheritance that is already ours.

And in believing the lie, we learn to settle for a story too small for us.

The Power of a Too-Small Story

If our lives aren't evidence enough, Scripture itself offers tale after tale of people inhabiting stories too small for them. Take Isaiah 30, for example. King Hezekiah is on the throne, having restored a kingdom nearly ruined by his father, Ahaz, a man whose inner storms wreaked havoc wherever he went, wounding the people of God. Hezekiah, whose name means "God has strengthened," loves God, and his own secure love manifests in reforms that strengthen the kingdom, restoring dignity, relationship, and purpose. It is said that "there was no one like him among all the kings of Judah, either before him or after him" (2 Kings 18:5). He restores the Temple where God dwells and reinstates the festivals in order to remember God's goodness and the nation's deep union and communion with God. He calls his people to remember the better story, the story of God's *hesed*—his extravagant loving-kindness. Hezekiah is living freely and fully within the big and beautiful story of God.

That is, until anxiety overwhelms him. With the daunting prospect of imminent invasion by the Assyrian armies to the north, good king Hezekiah panics. In his ear are military advisors whispering words of fear, escalating the threat. And they sell him and his advisors on a surefire strategy to cope. Hezekiah, instead of trusting in the one who brought such goodness, succumbs to the overwhelm of a Sympathetic Storm within. To cope, he grasps like Adam and Eve, and he enters into a security pact with Egypt, the nation that had enslaved God's people many centuries before. Instead of resting in the secure love he's come to know, his body remembers his own father's anxious and insecure clutching, no doubt familiar to him and even a part of his own story. He listens to the ancient voice of the serpent, which drowns out God's whisper of secure care and abiding presence. The power of an old, smaller story from the past takes hold, even in the great King Hezekiah.

In Egypt, of course, Hezekiah's ancestors experienced the slow erosion of their God-imaged identity. The indignity of a life of slavery ravaged them, and it took generations to restore their sense of worth, belonging, and purpose. Here now, even Hezekiah has forgotten the centuries-long faithfulness of God. Caught up in his own anxiety and insecurity, he fails to recall the larger story of goodness and grace. His body remembers a different narrative, a multigenerational history of pain and sabotage, a story his father had lived so recklessly, a story with roots generations before in Egypt.

The prophet Isaiah doesn't mince words, reminding Hezekiah and his advisors that living in this smaller story won't bring peace but only more shame:

> "Woe to the obstinate children,"
> > declares the LORD,
> "to those who carry out plans that are not mine,
> > forming an alliance, but not by my Spirit,
> > heaping sin upon sin;

who go down to Egypt
    without consulting me;
who look for help to Pharaoh's protection,
    to Egypt's shade for refuge.
But Pharaoh's protection will be to your shame,
    Egypt's shade will bring you disgrace."

ISAIAH 30:1-3

Amidst storming anxiety, the reaction is not to trust but to fight, not connection but self-protection. It's a reaction of insecurity, manifesting in sabotage and shame. Isaiah's words of caution and danger are for those "who make an alliance" (Isaiah 30:1, ESV), a verb in the Hebrew text that alludes to weaving a covering, even a security blanket,[1] recalling the fig leaves Adam and Eve gathered to cover themselves. Egypt was once a refuge for God's people during a time of famine, a temporary security blanket amidst a time of uncertainty. I can't help but think that Isaiah is warning his beloved friends not to get stuck in the past, not to return to the old and tattered blanket of Egypt's faux protection.

But Israel's old story holds power for them, and it comes roaring back, even in a time of plenty.

It's not hard to relate. Indeed, we've all experienced this. In such times, we might say that we're triggered—or, as I prefer, *activated*—as an old underlying memory or event surges into the present moment, our bodies charged with anxiety. It seems that in an instant we lose track of our deepest memory of worth, belonging, and purpose. As in the days of Hezekiah, things may be going quite well. Your marriage is good. Your job is satisfying. But something ignites the old voice of the serpent as you descend into doubt, self-contempt, insecurity, or shame, eventually grasping for something to soothe the ache. Perhaps your spouse fails to call you when they said they would, eliciting old feelings of abandonment. Or a fender bender activates a distant memory of being in a terrifying car accident as a child. Maybe a sense of disrespect from a boss sends you spiraling in shame. You thought you were over these things, beyond being so easily activated. But in an instant, you're right back there. And like the Israelites—and like Adam and Eve before them—you abandon the big and beautiful story of goodness, joy, and connection you were made for, returning instead to your old security blankets.

It's into this frazzling and frustrating place that God comes.

The Art of Redemptive Remembering

When my daughters, Emma and Maggie, were little, I'd rock them to sleep whispering goodness over them.

You are a delight. You are safe. You are loved.

In these tender moments, I prayed that the secure connection Sara and I were cultivating with our girls would accompany them amidst the inevitable challenges they'd experience as they grew up and ventured out. And I prayed that amidst our inconsistencies as parents, they'd know, at their core, that they were loved.

This is the tenderness God brings to the Garden. This is the love he brings to Adam and Eve, broken and hiding. God meets them in their suffering. He asks, "Where are you?" (Genesis 3:9), tenderly approaching them even as they hide, inviting them to wake up, to be seen, as hard as it is. God continues his probing: "Who told you?" (verse 11). He's inviting them to do something they'd perhaps rather not do—to recall where they've been, to reckon with the voices they've been listening to apart from God's, to remember who they are.

Even when the prophet Isaiah explains to Hezekiah and the Israelites the traumatic toll their choice will take, he can't help but remind them of God's kind invitation amidst it, saying, "In repentance and rest is your salvation, in quietness and trust is your strength" (Isaiah 30:15).

And this invitation to remember is ours today. In our shame and alienation, we expect God's summons to be harsh and punitive. Instead, we find it curious and compassionate.

"Who told you?" God asks in Genesis 3. What story are you listening to? Whose voice are you trusting? It's an invitation to reflect on our own stories, on the patterns we learned in our early schools of formation, even in our first years. It's an invitation to listen for the deeper story that God whispers over us still, the story God enters into history to enact, the story that compels God to come nearer still, by the Spirit, so that we can live free, full, and flourishing lives. Remembering reconnects us—to ourselves, to each other, to God.

It's not easy: We'll have to retrace our steps, asking hard questions, identifying the lies that ensnared us, perhaps even naming those within our story responsible for the lies. But this kind of redemptive remembering—where we once again recall our deep dignity and worth, our sense of connection and belonging, our call and purpose—can help us sift through our stories and begin to recognize where we've heard the serpent's lies. Even when we feel like we've messed up, God's kindness and compassion are never far. We can recall, even in our worst moments, that God's heart is *for* us, gently inviting us back Home. We can listen afresh to the voice of the One who is always secure, who can always be trusted—the One who calls us beloved.

Minding Our Own Stories

Within a few weeks of my wife, Sara, giving birth to our first daughter, Emma, I dropped her. Twice.

If you choose to keep reading on from here, I'm grateful.

On the first occasion, Sara was resting, and I was proudly in charge. I prepared to do a solo diaper change, not on the changing table in Emma's bedroom but on the ottoman, within view of our television and a football game I was watching. The large ottoman was wide and soft, holding Emma's small body comfortably as I looked away and reached for a diaper. In an instant, she somehow rolled off the ottoman, landing face down on the carpeted floor. She cried. I cried. I lifted her and held her, my self-punishing thoughts so loud and my body so activated that it took a bit to get back to center and start again.

A good dad would've known not to take my eyes off her, even for a minute.

You need to be more responsible.

You're not cut out for parenting.

On the second occasion, Sara and I had gone out to eat for the first time with Emma. We sat outdoors at a small Italian restaurant near our home. I again took charge, rocking our daughter to sleep and then laying her gently in her car seat. I set the handle back in place—but not all the way, for fear that the loud click of the handle's lock would wake her.

Thirty minutes later when we'd paid the bill and risen to leave the table, I grabbed the car seat by the unlocked handle. I felt the whole thing shift, and again, in an instant, Emma fell face down, this time onto a concrete outdoor deck. She cried. I shrunk in shame. Sara quickly picked Emma up and comforted her. And I nearly resigned from parenting. I thought I'd failed.

I'd felt so ready to be a dad. When I was working on my counseling graduate degree in seminary, I studied John Bowlby's attachment theory, that groundbreaking work that shows how our earliest relationships with caregivers forge our sense of self, mapping our style of relating and social engagement for the rest of our lives. It was through this that I began to recognize my own attachment style, manifesting in insecurity and anxiety. I wondered, at times, if I was really lovable, if I was enough, if I really belonged. And I tried to work on healing my own wounds so that I wouldn't wound my kids.

I wanted to do everything I could to make sure we provided what Bowlby called "secure" attachment, assuring that Emma was safe, seen, soothed, and secure.[2] I read and readied myself. I did my own therapeutic work. But after two drops, I wasn't so sure Emma was safe with me. If I couldn't be trusted to keep her upright, how could I be trusted to guide her in this world?

Professors Todd and M. Elizabeth Lewis Hall write, "Memories of relational experiences with emotionally significant people are etched in our souls and become filters that shape how we feel about ourselves, God, and others, and how we determine the meaning of events in our lives."[3] Obviously, I don't really believe now that dropping Emma (twice) has shaped her so fundamentally. There is a lot in the stew of our parenting, some good and some not so good. We stumble. We fail. It's inevitable. While Sara and I did a lot of the right things, we still brought our imperfect selves and our unfinished stories into our parenting.

That's because the stories that shaped us keep re-storying in our adult lives. We're formed in the crucible of early parental attachments. Not only do we bear the inherited trauma of our parents and grandparents, but we also inherit the maps of how they attached to their caregivers.[4]

There are four primary attachment styles, and as the Halls suggest, exploring how your experience fits within each can be very important. However, I invite you to take this a step further. I believe each attachment style either supports or erodes our God-imaged sense of worth, belonging, and purpose. And understanding which attachment style resonates with our experience—understanding our stories—can help us discover how our earliest relationships have shaped our current relationships to ourselves, to each other, even to God.[5]

Now, the danger with attachment styles is the same as the danger with personality testing—we're always looking for the one thing to explain everything about us. Instead, I invite you to see these as lenses, a way of answering God's second question by remembering your own story, naming your patterns, and discovering how the serpent's lie might be showing up in your current sense of worth, belonging, and purpose. Seeing attachment in this way will help you become less concerned with labels, free to become curious about your story and to heal what's within.

Secure attachment

Jamie came to see me for counseling amidst a challenging season of losing both of her aging parents to Covid-19 within a month. She grieved that she couldn't see them in the end, as they were quarantined in their assisted living facility. And yet, through tears and a smile of delight, she said, "But I've always felt seen by them. And I couldn't be more grateful for a love that I've never, ever doubted."

Secure attachment is the safe haven we all long for. Secure attachment offers the embodied experience of the kind of connection we were created to have, reminding us of our worth and securing our sense of belonging, even anchoring us to a sense of meaning and purpose in the world. In a sense, a caregiver echoes what God has already imprinted in the child as an image bearer. There are at least five conditions that allow this to happen:[6]

- *Safety:* The caregiver conveys safety by holding, comforting, protecting, feeding, and soothing their child. Safety is an echo of the relational intimacy of Eden, held and loved in the compassionate embrace of God.

- *Attunement:* The caregiver relationally sees and knows their child. They consistently sense their child's signals and respond in moments of need. Attunement is an echo of our intrinsic connection to God, who walks with us, sees us, and knows us.
- *Regulation:* The caregiver senses distress in their child and provides their own stable, non-anxious presence to help the child regulate. Regulation is an echo of the profound security we experience in God.
- *Delight:* The caregiver offers joy, affection, and a sense of deep worth to their child, which allows the child to internalize that sense of feeling loved and enjoyed. Delight is an echo of God's whisper of goodness and worth over us.
- *Authenticity:* The caregiver gives their child room to explore the world within the safety of their care. This allows the child to emerge into their own unique self. Authenticity is an echo of God's call on each of us to become ourselves, living with our own individual sense of purpose as image bearers.

Amidst the secure attachment offered by safe and attuned parents, a child develops into an adult who is capable of both connection to others and differentiation from others; that is, they know how to move in and out of relationships healthily and with appropriate boundaries.

Of course, securely attached people are not exempt from trauma. However, they are more anchored in their God-created sense of worth, more apt to have healthy relationships, and more connected to a personal sense of meaning, call, and purpose. They are less likely to self-soothe in addiction, cope with distraction, even plummet into depression. To be sure, they can't avoid the challenges of life. Storms will come. The Fog will envelop. But they are anchored in their Home, resourced internally to navigate the inevitable weather patterns that come their way.

Preoccupied (anxious) attachment

Ben was distraught as he entered my office, heartbroken that his fiancée had ended their engagement. Dani had grown weary of Ben's jealousy, his clinginess, and his lack of any friendships outside of her. "I'm nothing. I have no one. I'm all alone, and I'll always be alone," he said.

As we've seen, children need the secure connection a parent can offer. A parent won't offer this perfectly, but ideally a child comes to expect that their parent will be there consistently. In a preoccupied (anxious) attachment style, it is this consistency that is missing. The terrifying trauma of being alone and abandoned will activate their survival-based nervous system, prompting a desperate search for the soothing waters of connection, be it with the parent or, in their absence, a more unhealthy pseudo-connection with another adult.

As these children grow up, they frequently face ongoing struggles with anxiety. Operating from the script of preoccupied attachment, they often become hypervigilant as adults, always aware of the possibility of connection and rejection, ever alert to the latter. As Krispin Mayfield describes in his excellent work *Attached to God*, those whose stories were shaped in anxious attachment are preoccupied with their lack of worth and insecure in God's love. Their way of remaining connected to God may be performative, and they may chase emotional highs, only to find themselves feeling alone and unloved. Terrified of abandonment and unable to regulate the painful emotions that can often flood them, they find ways to stay close to those who they think will love them, even at the expense of their disowned needs. They're prone to misread relationships, oversharing with someone who isn't safe or trusting someone who is untrustworthy; almost inevitably, they find themselves in retraumatizing relationships, where real or perceived rejection happens again.

Lacking their image-bearing sense of inherent worth, deep belonging, and clear purpose, they try to secure their sense of worth on the outside, grasping for any breadcrumb of connection. Their strategy to survive looks a lot like a Storm: They may elicit angry demands (*fight*), withdraw manipulatively (*flight*), feign cooperation (*fawn*), or desperately grasp at connection (*find*). When those strategies don't work, they'll either become ambivalently paralyzed (*freeze*) or give up by completely shutting off their desire (*fold*).[7] Perpetually misattuned, they may become further and further frustrated with themselves, unknowingly magnifying their own pain. This can result in a wearying cycle of hypoarousal and hyperarousal, a never-ending hamster wheel of dysregulation and disconnection, and thus enduring trauma.

Dismissive (avoidant) attachment

Janet started counseling for the first time in her fifties after her staff at a Christian nonprofit confronted her for being a distant, detached, and unempathetic leader. She was puzzled by their grievances. "I didn't need to be fussed over like these young people do today," she told me. "I've always been happy just getting to work, putting my head down, and staying in my own lane. Needy people just slow you down."

Whereas the anxious attachment style is defined by emotional *inconsistency* of the caregiver, the dismissive/avoidant attachment style is defined by emotional *unavailability*. In adulthood, those with this attachment style are dismissive of relational and emotional needs—and thus dismissive of the connection for which they have been created. When they read a book like this, they may shrug their shoulders at the continual call to spiritual and emotional connection. As one of my clients said, "I'm just not wired that way." But this disconnected and dismissive state is not about wiring. In fact, attachment and temperament have very little in common.[8] Instead, it's a childhood story re-storied throughout a lifetime, a defensive wall erected to protect themselves from pain. Deep inside the walls, however, is someone who longs to be seen and who is hungry for a sense of worth, connection, and purpose.

Though someone with dismissive attachment seems less anxious than someone with preoccupied attachment, they are no less dysregulated. They may bully others with no sense of their impact (*fight*), avoid engagement altogether (*flight*), dispassionately appease (*fawn*), or strive for some sort of truce (*find*). When those strategies don't work, they'll either become numbly disconnected (*freeze*) or altogether unavailable (*fold*), manifesting in emotional shutdown, blunted emotion, an isolated disposition, and an averted gaze, which is thought to originate from the self-protective avoidance of disgust on a caregiver's face.[9] While those who are preoccupied overshare, those who are dismissive don't share. When asked for a feeling, they may offer a thought. And when invited to become curious about why they relate the way they do, they're apt to lack curiosity.[10] If their family story comes up, they will likely report a good childhood, but they won't have access to a coherent narrative about it. They have trouble remembering their story. And they are radically out of touch with who and whose they really are, at their core.

As you might expect, this distant and disconnected state is mapped onto their posture toward God, manifesting in a heady and rigid engagement. They settle for a very left-brained, logical way of relating to God, often finding their way to faith traditions that jettison emotion in favor of information. But while it may be tempting to think that the best way to help is through a book or better information, it's actually connection they need. Behind the walls is someone who longs to feel safe, seen, soothed, and secure.[11]

Fearful (disorganized) attachment

After she had broken a final boundary, Gina's roommates asked her to move out, prompting her to cope by cutting and binge drinking. She came to her counseling appointment with me late, hungover, and disheveled. "You'll probably kick me out too," she blurted within the first minute. "I manage to ruin any good relationship I have."

When we combine the inconsistency of anxious attachment and the unavailability of avoidant attachment, we get fearful or disorganized attachment. What seems to be true of those who are fearfully attached in adulthood is that they experienced a kind of complex, developmental form of trauma in childhood. Here we should recognize that kids who are abused are often raised by parents who also experienced abuse, a tragic multigenerational story that keeps on re-storying. The fearful and disorganized attachment style of the parent is mapped onto the child.[12]

While the fairly predictable styles of preoccupation and avoidance seem to make sense to most, the fearful (disorganized) attachment style can be confusing. This is because it is profoundly confusing for those who experience it. They don't trust themselves. They don't trust you. They want love, and they reach for it. They know love will hurt, and they pull back. They are mired in shame. It's a maddening internal reality for many. Most suffer alone, struggling to attend to what's happening within. This is because there is an internal game of ping-pong that has them bouncing between Storm and Fog in order to survive. They live in constant disorientation. Parts of them feel at war with one another, and they can simultaneously feel broken beyond repair and suspicious of anyone trying to help, believing that people are out to harm them. Even in therapeutic work, good opportunities for real care can be sabotaged, not intentionally but as a trauma response. At times, self-harm is the only path of soothing they can find.[13]

Here in this traumatic terrain, a God-created sense of worth, belonging, and purpose may seem like a fairy tale that will never be theirs. The faith story they live within is filled with shame and terror, their sense of God not as curious or compassionate but as punitive, doubling down on their shame and self-contempt. They may idealize a pastor or faith community at first, hopeful that this is where they'll finally find love. But their idealism may quickly flip to cynicism and self-protection when they perceive a lack of safety. Indeed, they long for love, but they walk in a world filled with emotional land mines threatening their sense of security.

That said, if and when they discover the beauty of secure relationships and learn to trust, despite internal promptings to sabotage, they can experience deep repair and healing at both a neurobiological and relational level. Indeed, many often begin to marvel at God's patient, attuned care, even amidst their doubts and detours.

● ● ●

Perhaps you, like me, find yourself relating to more than one attachment style. The reality is that you were formed and shaped in a matrix of relationships, and you likely act differently in different contexts and relationships. Some people find that there is a primary attachment style they resonate with, but many notice ways of relating that match more than one attachment style. I can personally see aspects of an anxious attachment with my mother and an avoidant attachment with my father. This manifests in a mixed map for my present relationships, as my wife, Sara, is all too familiar with!

Yet, as you better understand your attachments, you can turn your attention to your current relationships, noticing how your childhood stories are re-storied in your patterns of relating today. Attachments can offer a window into the smaller stories you get stuck in, helping you to name what you needed, what was missing, what happened, and where you were wounded—for by remembering in this way, you remember how to return Home.

Attachment science reminds us that the past need not repeat itself in the present. There is great hope. Your attachment wounds can find healing in your present-day relationships, where you can be reminded of who you really are. Though you might be experiencing a form of insecure attachment, growth and healing are possible. By building secure relationships and investing in healthy church, work, and social environments, you can experience what attachment psychologists call "earned secure attachment."[14] I'd prefer to call this *realized secure attachment*. You can't acquire or earn what is already yours, but you can realize that, at your core, you are the beloved and that worth, belonging, and purpose are your inheritance as an image bearer. You can recognize that your deepest self is "hidden with Christ in God" (Colossians 3:3) and not merely reconstructed in the matrix of relationships.

To realize this, however, you and I need communities of redemptive remembering, where we're invited to recall the story of God, where our own stories are welcomed in all their complexity, and where we're invited to remember who we are. We need communities where our wounds are welcomed, where our long-and-winding journeys Home are stewarded, and where we're known and loved.

Communities of redemptive remembering invite us out of the exile of Sympathetic Storm and Dorsal Fog, drawing us into a new family where we can experience peace, belonging, presence, dignity, and purpose (see Ephesians 2:11-22). In place of old, toxic understandings of God that were formed in the churning storm amidst insecure attachments, we can now experience his security, compassion, and kindness as he rewires us so we can feel his reliable motherly and fatherly embrace. Even amidst the trauma of insecure attachment, we can find our way Home.

The Practice of Redemptive Remembering

Things were going well for me in the years after we left San Francisco. Much of the Fog had cleared. But on a day of would-be celebration, my body revolted. I was up for tenure at the seminary where I teach, and there was no doubt I'd get it. But when I was asked to leave the gathering so that my colleagues could vote, shame started screaming within me, anxiety overwhelming my body. What was just minutes felt like hours. Within me, a torrent of voices, echoes of the slithering serpent, sent me spiraling into self-contempt. *They're in there talking about how laughable it is that you're up for this. They know better.*

You're not worth it. Make it easy for them and withdraw now. You know you're not wanted anyway. You know they're looking for a way to get you out of here.

My nervous system stormed within. I could barely catch my breath. I wondered where I could go to hide. I lost my sense of time, my episodic memory. Days later I only vaguely remembered how it all went down. Clearly, an old story of trauma was re-storying in me in that moment, taking me out of the joy and celebration of the present and tugging me back into my shame-riddled season of rejection.

When the dust settled and I came home to myself, I breathed deeply and received the gift of a practice I share with you on page 105. I imagined the face of Jesus, smiling, whispering, "I see you. I love you. You are my beloved. You belong." I began hearing within myself whispers of God's kindness, as Scriptures I'd read and heard over the years began coming to mind:

I long to make my face shine upon you and to be gracious to you.[15]
Nothing can separate you from my love.[16]
I am compassionate and gracious, slow to anger, abounding in love.[17]
You are always with me, and everything I have is yours.[18]

My body relaxed. I experienced a deep sense of goodness and rest, which allowed me to recall the goodness of that day. In my mind's eye, I saw my colleagues smiling and clapping. They welcomed me into a time-honored tradition of belonging. They prayed for me. Now at Home, my body re-membered, putting the pieces back together again.

Sometimes the call is to listen to the One whose voice is so much more kind than any other. Our centering practices, which include the one's we've already explored, allow us to rest and remember. But if we're unable to hear or if we're stuck for some reason, we may need to muster up the courage to ask for help, even therapeutic help, to get unstuck.

At least part of what we do in therapy is to create the conditions under which the body can safely re-member. When trauma disconnects and dismembers in ways that keep us from remembering and healing, mental health professionals have a number of ways of slowly and methodically re-accessing the frozen past. Through modalities like EMDR, Internal Family Systems (IFS), somatic therapies, and more, well-trained clinicians are able to engage the subcortical regions of the brain not accessible through traditional talk therapies.[19] Here, the work is slow, paced for your unique journey. But, where trauma disconnects different regions of the brain, these therapeutic techniques offer the possibility of reconnection and even retrieval of memories locked away. Slowly, we're re-membered, our lives and our bodies becoming more integrated, more whole. Perhaps you might discern whether or not you need to pursue a more structured, therapeutic journey for your healing.

Disregarding what's happening within you only keeps you stuck, alienated from your past, numbed in your present. And the helpful insights of contemporary psychology echo the wisdom of millennia—we remember and retell the story so that we don't get stuck going forward (Deuteronomy 8:2). As I've said at various times while leading people to the Communion table, "Some people drink to forget. We drink to remember." Some drink to numb the pain, to self-soothe amidst the wounds of life, even those that've gone unspoken. At the Communion table, however, we remember: In the presence of God, we remember what Christ has done for us, his body broken, his blood shed, a God wounded in order to heal us of our wounds. We remember where we've been—the dead-end roads and detours we've taken—as we come to a feast fit for our flourishing. Chewing on bread and sipping wine is an embodied act. Our bodies are implicated in God's mysterious means of putting us back together again, of re-membering us, amidst divisions within and without. At this table, our shattered shards are reconnected by the One whose body was broken for us. At this table, we're freed to live lives of wholeness, of shalom, going forward.

This beautiful mystery is a practice of redemptive remembering. This practice invites us to explore our stories but also to remember and be re-membered in *God's* story. And it's not lost on me that the same God who whispered, "Who told you?" came in the flesh, invited his beloved to a table for a feast, and invited them to remember too. God's pursuit of us is an invitation back to the oneness and worthiness we experienced in Eden, into a union and communion that makes us whole.

Henri Nouwen writes, "Our first and most important spiritual task is to claim God's unconditional love for ourselves. To remember who we truly are in the memory of God. . . . That we are God's beloved."[20] This is the deeper challenge of God's "Who told you?" In it, we hear God asking, "Whose voice are you listening to?" And we strain to hear, even amidst the lies of the serpent. This isn't easy. The lies get lodged deep within. Eventually, they may become the only story we tell ourselves.

But God gives us resources to restore us. God gives us tables to remember around. God gives us people to remind us. And God gives us the invitation to remember who we truly are, that we are his beloved. May we remember and be re-membered.

RESOURCES

- Dan B. Allender, *To Be Told: Know Your Story, Shape Your Future*
- Frederick Buechner, *Telling Secrets*
- Janina Fisher, *Transforming the Living Legacy of Trauma: A Workbook for Survivors and Therapists*
- Todd W. Hall, *The Connected Life: The Art and Science of Relational Spirituality*
- Henri Nouwen, *The Return of the Prodigal Son: A Story of Homecoming*

Reflection

1. How does Hezekiah's story help you recognize the importance of exploring your own story? What aspects of Hezekiah's situation can you relate to?

2. The challenges of life can chip away at our God-imaged inheritance of worth, belonging, and purpose. We can become mired in shame, stuck in aloneness and isolation, trapped in disillusionment. Use the following questions to reflect on this:

- Who in my story championed my worth and belonging, and called me to a sense of purpose? What particular memories of hearing these messages from someone can you recall? What was spoken? How did it feel?

- Whose words shattered these things, prompting shame, alienation, and disillusionment? Is there a core story or stories you recall around this?

- Are there people in your life today who speak words of goodness, kindness, and compassion to you? How? What can you do to assure that there are people in your life who do see your image-bearing self and speak words of dignity, love, and vision for your flourishing? What fears do you have about this?

3. Which attachment styles help put words to your own story and how you tend to relate to others even today? Can you identify particular attachment "wounds" that have rendered you more preoccupied, dismissive, or fearful/shameful in your relationships with others or

with God? How does it help to understand that these aren't fixed personality styles but are patterns that can be changed through healing relationships and healthy communities? If there are others you are journeying with as you read this book, invite their feedback about how you relate and discuss what intentional things you might do to begin to heal.

Practice: Redemptive Remembering

Timeline exercise

Create a timeline for a particular season of your life (for example, your childhood and adolescence, or your late teens and early twenties). Draw a line across the middle of the page. Above the line, recall and record moments and stories when you experienced being seen and known as an image bearer; when your worth, belonging, and sense of purpose were affirmed. Below the line, record experiences, events, or words that tore away at these things, manifesting in shame, isolation, loneliness, anxiety, hopelessness, and self-protective strategies just to survive. For each section, see if you can pinpoint how these experiences unfolded, along with where, when, and with whom. Which experiences or events feel particularly pivotal in your sense of self-understanding? If you want to go deeper, consider engaging in this exercise with a therapist or a friend and share particular stories around it.

Imaginative re-storying

In this practice, you recall the story of God through the words of God, taken from whatever places in Scripture speak to you. You can draw on a variety of different passages, gathering them for this exercise. You might consider one of the following:

- Psalm 139:1-18
- Song of Songs 2
- John 15:1-17
- 1 Corinthians 6:19-20
- Galatians 5:13-26
- Ephesians 3:14-21

Now find an image, whether through a work of art or in your own imagination, of the face of Jesus, kind and compassionate and present. Wrap your arms across your chest in a butterfly hug and begin tapping, slowly and rhythmically. This motion is soothing and will also reconnect your often disconnected left and right brains. Make sure you're breathing, too, according to the guidance offered in chapter 1 (see pages 29–30). Now, read or listen to the words from those Scriptures. Hear them spoken over you. Enjoy the delight of being reminded of who you are and whose you are. Delight in God being with you. You may want to read or listen to them several times.

SAY HELLO

How We Cultivate the Most Healing Conversation
We May Ever Have

*I had awakened to a growing darkness and cacophony, as if
something in my depths were crying out. A whole chorus of voices.
Orphaned voices. They seemed to speak for all the unlived parts of me,
and they came with a force and dazzle that I couldn't contain.
They seemed to explode the boundaries of my existence. I know now
that they were the clamor of a new self struggling to be born.*

SUE MONK KIDD

"Hello there, little guy," I said. "Do you want to sit up front with me?"

I was driving home on a warm Tuesday morning in the Bay, and I'll admit, I was feeling a little silly. After all, I was talking to myself.

As part of an exercise given to me by my therapist, Jay, I was attempting to connect with the many parts of myself I'd learned to ignore over the years. Like many of us, I learned early on in life that more vulnerable parts of me weren't necessarily welcome, that it'd be better to toughen up than to tuck tail.

These tougher parts of me, Jay asserted, were just attempting to help me survive in a traumatic world, to protect those sensitive parts from getting hurt again. And, boy, did they work hard. I cordoned off every other part within that felt fragile or vulnerable. Instead, a part of me armored up with knowledge, ready to fight anyone who questioned my views. Another part of me remained perpetually cautious, always alert to the danger around me. Yet another part learned to play the game of people-pleasing and appeasing.

As an adult, the strong, survival-based, self-protective parts of me served a purpose; they kept the ship afloat in the years after I was fired. Like the serpent, these parts whispered within me, *Get it on your own, Chuck.* And I did. I put my competencies and intellect to good use earning a living and getting a PhD. I doubled down in San Francisco, working harder and making sure I produced. On the outside I looked smart, competent, and even emotionally healthy most of the time.

But on the inside, everything was out of order.

So in therapy, Jay didn't praise the parts of me that were competent, productive, and invulnerable, as some had in the past. Instead, he looked at me with compassion in his eyes. "They must be exhausted," he said. Indeed, he was right. Although it seemed as if he were channeling ancient wisdom, Jay was guided by a contemporary model for healing our warring passions within called Internal Family Systems (IFS). We worked to turn toward every part of myself with a gaze of kindness and curiosity, even with a kind "hello." Each part had a story—a burden, a wound suffered alone within. And each offered me the invitation to redemptively remember, as the shattered shards within began to mend, as I became more whole.

And that little guy in the proverbial front seat? He was terrified.

When he was young, he'd hide under a side table in his living room, sometimes curling into a ball, hoping to become invisible. He couldn't quite remember all the details. But he knew it was the safest place to be when his mom was angry or when his parents were fighting.

He was a tenderhearted kid, the kind who could sense a storm brewing before it even arrived, a barometer for human relationships. He sensed the incoming weather, felt it in the shifting tones of his mother's voice and how loudly she'd bang the pots and pans while loading the dishwasher. And when he was little, that side table was never far from view. But he remained cloistered even as the years passed, always peeking around the corner, ever aware of the condescending tone of a boss, always sensitive to the anxious air in every room.

So as I continued my drive that Tuesday, I tried again. "Hello there, little guy," I said, casting off my self-consciousness and leaning into the exercise Jay had encouraged. "Do you want to sit up front with me?"

He did. As we drove, I asked him if he was glad to be out from under the side table. After all, the house he grew up in has been completely renovated and has a new owner. He smiled. He was happy to be free. But he reported that he'd always traveled with me, always remained within, cloaked in darkness, ever afraid, suffering alone.

"Don't leave me again," he said.

"I'm here with you now," I whispered back. "And so is Jesus."

I sensed him looking at me with a big smile and bright eyes. Thrilled at the chance to sit alongside me in the convertible Mini Cooper I'd recently bought, we left the foothills of Mount Tam, cruising back through the Rainbow Tunnel, top down, the vast red expanse of the Golden Gate Bridge ahead. He threw his hands in the air and shouted "Woooooo!" as we crossed.

The fog was clearing.

All the Scattered Feelings Within

Disney Pixar's 2015 movie *Inside Out* might just be the most helpful movie I've ever seen for the work I do. The trailer sounds the invitation to "meet the little voices inside your head,"[1] the voices of joy, fear, disgust, anger, sadness, and more. It follows the story of Riley, an eleven-year-old coping with her family's cross-country move. As you might imagine, her joyful preteen life is disrupted in the process. And the animated film offers an inside look at the disruption, showing her emotions personified as parts of her with their own unique personalities, needs, and longings, all of which begin to war within and without.

It's a movie that dignifies all these emotions. Joy brings happiness and connection. Anger seeks fairness. Fear offers safety. Disgust looks out for her in social situations. And Sadness, as we discover, seeks help and care. But in the overwhelm of a move, different parts vie for control. Joy spins everything as positive, ignoring the pain. Anger rages. Disgust alienates. Fear panics. And Sadness is exiled. Riley's capacity to navigate it all well is contingent on these parts finding their way back to connection with her and with each other, of these parts being re-membered.

I read that the producers of the film worked behind the scenes with psychologists and neuroscientists to understand the role of emotion and memory. But the kids watching it won't be confused by the science of it all. No, they might just learn to listen within, to give voice to sadness or fear, to allow anger to speak without taking over, to say hello even to shame and disgust. I remember watching it with tears in my eyes, thinking especially of my sweet and tenderhearted daughter Maggie, who'd taken our move from San Francisco to Michigan especially hard, whose own sadness, anger, and fear mirrored Riley's.

"Trauma is when we are not seen and known," says Bessel van der Kolk.[2] And what both *Inside Out* and ancient wisdom teachers might agree on is that we need a compassionate witness to our pain. Absent this, parts of us go it on their own, as we become more and more disoriented and disconnected, alienated from ourselves, one another, and God. Here, we're lonely and lost, wounded and wandering. And if we don't recognize the disorder within and get the care we need, we'll only become more divided within. Trauma expert Janina Fisher names the tax of remaining strangers to ourselves:

> Over time, self-alienation can only be maintained by most individuals at the cost of increasingly greater self-loathing, disconnection from emotion, addictive or self-destructive behavior, and internal struggles

between vulnerability and control, love and hate, closeness and distance, shame and pride.[3]

Disordered within and disconnected from the Love who whispers to us from our deepest core, we get stuck in chronic fight or flight, in codependent fawning and desperate grasping to find the supposed love we need. Our internal Storms become the only reality we know. I now see how I lived a self-alienated existence, playing an exhausting game of emotional Whac-A-Mole for too long. Many of us do. Numbing and distracting can work for a surprisingly long time.

Is Something Wrong with Me?

I wish I'd had *Inside Out* to watch when things began falling apart for me in the summer of 1997.

I was studying in Oxford, England, doing my best to write weekly term papers in order to secure my tutor's recommendation for a doctoral program in New Testament studies. While it might not sound like your ideal summer, it was a mid-twenty-something seminary student's dream. Days in the Bodleian Library. Evenings at The Eagle and Child Pub. I was in the land of C. S. Lewis and J. R. R. Tolkien. It should have been the best of times.

But for me, it was a land mired in Sympathetic Storm. My anxious body began to conspire against me even then, the pressure of impressing my tutor and gaining his recommendation taxing my body and soul. Panic would seize me during our sessions together, my mouth dry, my heart thumping, my hands shaking. I'd walk away beating myself up for being so stupid, so messed up. It seemed as if my future hinged on this one person's approval of me—and I was bombing it, or so I thought. For five weeks, I endured a cycle of anticipatory anxiety, panic, and then disgust, all chased away by a few hard ciders at night. I returned home to the States exhausted and sick, my weary body beleaguered.

With little sense of how it would help, I had the good intuition to book a meeting with Gary, our seminary counseling professor. Like a perceptive doctor of the soul, Gary read the script of my life like a book, offering me kindness and care— my very first human experience of God's "Where are you?" He recommended a local therapist, and I promptly booked my first appointment. But after a couple of relatively helpful sessions, I noticed a numerical code and some small print on the receipt with the name of my mental-health disorder.

Disorder?

With little understanding of what was going on within me and without a movie like *Inside Out* to help, I spiraled into self-contempt. I read my diagnosis like a disease I'd been plagued with. Disorder seemed to name my deepest me. And I *hated* the disordered me. Hadn't I worked so hard to appear perfectly ordered? I looked around at my seminary peers, who appeared so put together, and my disgust for my own screwed-up self grew.

Mind you, I'd been schooled in self-contempt prior to this; a student of a simplified, flannelgraph faith, I grew up believing disorder was core to who I was, that I was *defined* more by my sin than by God's declaration of my deep worth, belonging, and purpose. And it stuck. This is the experience of many—questions about our worth and goodness begin at a very early age, and it's a well-known psychological truism that children believe themselves to be bad to protect themselves from the reality that others, including their parents, are flawed and fallible. "It's my fault," we reckon, even before we have the capacity to reason it through.

By my late teen years, purely because of my existence in the world, I believed I was bad to the core. And though I believed that Jesus had died to save me from my sins, that theological truth didn't seem to touch my core experience of badness. I prayed for God to root out all the badness in me. Now, a decade later, my psychological diagnosis was proof to me that those prayers had gone unanswered.

No one ever told me that this was a version of the serpent's lie. What I didn't grasp years ago that I see much better today is that *disorder* isn't so much about *the very bad thing wrong with you to the core* as much as things within being *not in the right order.* They are out of order. Just as they were in the movie.

Inside Out in the Story of God

St. Augustine called sin disordered love; that is, that there is something going on within us that isn't core to us, but that certainly is disrupting, disorienting, and disordering us. "Now if I do what I do not want to do," Paul writes, "it is no longer I who do it, but it is sin living in me that does it" (Romans 7:20). On the one hand, we know we're image bearers, delighted in at our core, but we're also quite aware of how far we've strayed from center, disconnected from our deepest identity. We all feel it. It seems as if parts of us take over, overwhelming us, steering the ship in the wrong direction. You begin to sense the dis-order in Paul's own autobiographical account in Romans 7. He writes, "I do not understand what I do. For what I want to do I do not do, but what I hate I do" (7:15).

Seeking to understand himself, Augustine describes this feeling viscerally: "I am scattered. . . . Storms of incoherent events tear to pieces my thoughts, the inmost entrails of my soul."[4] And this is what disorder feels like, doesn't it? It tears us away from Home, pulling us into Storm and Fog, marring our ability to see clearly. We begin to feel as if we're losing connection with ourselves. We lose the plot of God's good story.

This is exactly how I felt in Oxford. Different parts of me were vying for control. Fear would take the wheel, driving with extreme vigilance, making sure I was dotting all of my academic *i*'s and crossing all of my performative *t*'s to secure a tutor's approval. A bit of healthy fear might've allowed me to mobilize well for the work, but this inordinate panic exhausted me. Weary after a long day, another part of me would take over. He sought soothing, mostly in food, drink, and distracting conversation. And these weren't the only players in my inner drama.

In the New Testament, James warns that, left unattended, these wars within will inevitably leak out, manifesting in relational conflict. He offers the helpful language of "passions":

What causes fights and what causes quarrels among
you? Is it not this, that your passions are at war within

you? You desire and do not have, so you murder. You
covet and cannot obtain, so you fight and quarrel. You
do not have, because you do not ask. You ask and do
not receive, because you ask wrongly, to spend it on
your passions.

JAMES 4:1-3 (MY PARAPHRASE)

Others in the early church resonated with James's language
of passions. The desert mothers and fathers—women and men
who left their homes in order to better live at peace with God
and each other—sat in silence in order to better hear the warring passions (Latin for "suffering") within. They described
what was happening with terms like *fear* and *envy*, *pride* and
gluttony, *lust* and *greed*, *anger* and *sloth*; all words to name the
shifting emotions within us. It was an early church version of
Inside Out. Theologian Wendy Farley writes,

> The "passions" is an ancient name for some of the ways
> in which our own psyche helps to trap us in patterns of
> living that block us from our deepest joy. . . . Passions
> have the connotation of bondage and uneasiness.
> They exemplify the way the soul can become twisted
> and turned in on itself and alienated from the world
> around us.[5]

Ordinary and good emotions can become chronic states of
suffering. Yet, while the desert mothers and fathers—and Paul
and Augustine too—wrote intimately of this inner tug-of-war,

these passions, and this disorder within, they didn't see it as core to who we truly are as children of God. As Farley describes, it's not that the passions of fear or lust *are* us; rather, they take control of us in a way that disconnects us from our deepest selves, in a way that makes us feel we are defined by our disorder. I suspect that was always the goal of that slithering serpent in Genesis 3.

Our work, then, is to listen for the echoes of this lie in our own stories so that we can return back to our original design. Back to Home. God's image in you and me speaks to our inherent worth, intimate belonging, and profound purpose. It's because God sees us *whole* and not as a hopeless collection of disordered parts that we can be re-membered, restored, reconnected to Love. It's because God's memory of us runs deeper than our own that we can find our way back Home, that we can be found, each of us a hungry and heartsick prodigal. It's because God goes after us—even when we're turned inside out—that we can experience freedom and flourishing.

God's pursuit begins just as soon as we lose track of ourselves. As Adam and Eve hide behind fig leaves, anxious and ashamed, God meets them, whispering, "Where are you? Who told you?" God sees through the fig leaves. God knows your deepest you because God designed your deepest you for goodness, beauty, and freedom. Dwelling within, God invites you back in union and communion. Augustine writes, "Lo, you were within, but I outside, seeking there for you. . . . You were with me, but I was not with you."[6] God is your compassionate witness, your guiding beacon from within leading every weary and wounded part of you back Home.

And it's this kindness, which God intends to turn you back to him (see Romans 2:4), that leads you on a journey of inner transformation. At its core, repentance (*metanoia*) is about a new way of seeing and living that invites an internal reordering, followed by a deeper connection to the One who delights in you.

Strangers Become Friends: Turning Inward with Compassion

The apostle Paul wrote, "I am convinced that nothing can ever separate us from God's love. Neither death nor life, neither angels nor demons, neither our fears for today nor our worries about tomorrow—not even the powers of hell can separate us from God's love" (Romans 8:38, NLT). Few people illustrate that truth more clearly than the gifted poet Pádraig Ó Tuama. Subjected to exorcisms as a young man in an attempt to set him straight and eventually exiled from the priesthood when they didn't take, he continued to search for healing. While he may well have spent the rest of his life warring against the church or even warring against himself, he turned his energies toward love. He'd been exiled. But God hadn't abandoned him.

And Ó Tuama lived into the truth that God was eager to greet him.

In his lovely work *In the Shelter*, he tells the story of a Taizé retreat he attended where a monk invited various attendees to read the biblical story of Jesus' appearance to the disciples in the upper room. The monk told his guests that Jesus greeted his disciples by saying, "Peace be with you." Ó Tuama tells the rest of the story:

The Taizé brother suggested that we pause for a moment and consider the words "Peace be with you" that the resurrected Jesus says to his locked-in followers. The Taizé brother said that, in a real sense, we can read that as "Hello." After all, it's the standard greeting in Hebrew, Arabic, and Aramaic. . . .

The disciples were there, in fear, in an upper room, locked away, and suddenly the one they had abandoned and perhaps the one they most feared to be with them was with them, and he said hello.

Hello to you in this locked room.[7]

Throughout the book, Ó Tuama employs the practice of greeting parts of himself and experiences within his story with a simple "hello."

Hello to the gift of being wrong.
Hello to the need for change.
Hello, distraction.
Hello, chaos.[8]

And through this practice, strangers within became friends. Parts relegated to the dungeons of his psyche came out to be healed. He discovered in this practice a kindness that would allow him to face every wounded and weary part of himself and to chart a course to wholeness.

No one said, however, that this course would be smooth.

Living Self-Compassionately

A client of mine named Jen realized this during our few years of work together. She came to me because of the work I was doing on narcissism in the church and, in large part, because she was raised as the daughter of a narcissistic pastor and now found herself married to one. She pinballed between fight and flight, warring against her husband in brutal fights or by cordoning herself off in a separate bedroom, sometimes not coming out for days.

The wars Jen couldn't win at home she waged on social media. Amidst her powerlessness, a part of her that felt powerful scrolled for hours, posting and challenging others, especially where she saw hypocrisy and abuse happening within the church. "Sometimes I just get caught up in the moment, and it's like this fierce side of me comes out that has never had a voice," she said during one session. And in many ways, I completely understood why she was doing this, feeling repulsed myself at the toxic spirituality she was calling out.

"I get it," I said to Jen. "And yet I'd also like to get to know the parts of you that feel powerless, defeated, even exhausted." She sat back and said, "You're the first person I've ever felt safe enough to share those parts of me with. It feels good to sit here and not have to be defensive. It feels safe enough to let you see how scared I really am."

Gabor Maté notes that if we continue to try to treat on the outside what is really a wound on the inside, we'll get nowhere. But if we can shift our gaze to the war going on within us, we can begin to heal:

Seeing trauma as an internal dynamic grants us much-needed agency. If we treat trauma as an external event, something that happens *to* or around us, then it becomes a piece of history we can never dislodge. If, on the other hand, trauma is what took place *inside* us as a result of what happened, in the sense of wounding or disconnection then healing and reconnection become tangible possibilities.[9]

Slowly, Jen began to make the shift to attending to what was happening within her. She shed tears for the relentless warrior part of her. *You don't have to fight so hard anymore,* she whispered within. *It's time to heal.*

She was beginning to do exactly what Ó Tuama suggests—she was compassionately greeting every wounded and weary part of herself:

Hello, raging social media warrior. It's time to rest.
Hello, frightened little girl. It's safe to share your hurt.

In time, Jen began to experience a new sense of strength—real power—a deep feeling of security in her experience of God's love and a deep feeling of safety that allowed for an inner re-ordering and integration to take place.

Rev. Martin Smith says it eloquently:

The Holy Spirit of God dwells in your heart and is no stranger to the diversity and conflict there. . . . There is no secret place where the Spirit has no access, nor any inner person excluded from the Spirit's presence. . . .

The Spirit will bring the selves of the self into a unity around the center of the indwelling Christ.[10]

Hello, Spirit. May the peace of Christ be in me and with me.

The Practice of Hello

Thomas Merton says, "To be born again is not to become somebody else, *but to become ourselves.*"[11] And don't you long to become yourself? Aren't you, like me, weary of coping, tired of surviving, worn-out from wearing the masks of all our other selves?

When we are able to turn inward with compassion—to greet the parts of us that long to come out of hiding—we move forward on the path of healing, of coming Home to ourselves. The practice of saying hello invites us to approach ourselves with the same compassion of God in Genesis 3, the same compassion Jesus offers when he says, "Peace be with you." Yes, the lies are loud within us. And it's easy to forget. But self-compassion, not self-condemnation, is the way forward. Curt Thompson says it well:

> Those parts of us that feel most broken and that we keep most hidden are the parts that most desperately need to be known by God, so as to be loved and healed. . . . God came to find Eve and Adam to provide

them the opportunity to be known as he knows
anything else. For only in those instances when our
shamed parts are known do they stand a chance to be
redeemed. We can love God, love ourselves or love
others only to the degree that we are known by God
and known by others.[12]

Offering this compassionate and even redemptive greeting
can be challenging. Jesus does not condemn the woman caught
in adultery in John 8, but he does call her Home, to reordered
love, to reconnection. And that road Home can be daunting,
as the lies of the serpent continue to echo within. That's why
the practice of hello will be a lifetime one for you. Around
every turn, you'll discover new ways in which you've grasped for
control or hidden parts of yourself away. And yet around every
turn, there God will be to greet you again.

Often the practice of hello needs to begin in relationship with a caring friend, an attuned pastor, a compassionate
therapist. At times you may need to sit with someone kind,
someone who can mirror your God-given worth, offering
you connection and care, courageously calling you to more,
before you can continue this practice on your own. You do
this through giving attention and attunement to parts of yourself that need care.

This is what I attempted to do as I continued the conversation while steering my convertible across the bridge:

Hello, little guy. You don't need to hide anymore.

You may need to acknowledge the hidden part of yourself at the business meeting when you stumble over your words and a fire surges up through your chest and into your face.

Hello, shame. I'm with you. It's okay.

Or perhaps after a surge of rage within, even after harsh words to a spouse or criticism of a coworker.

*Hello, rage. Take a deep breath. Let's find our way back
to center.*

Henri Nouwen writes, "Self-rejection is the greatest enemy of the spiritual life because it contradicts the sacred voice that calls us the 'Beloved.' Being the Beloved constitutes the core truth of our existence."[13] And while there are parts of you that you might be frustrated by, even parts that you might consider bad or broken to the core, you're invited to practice the same tenderness toward yourself that God offers you. Send them a kind hello, offering compassionate presence to whatever parts of you are activated within. It may be just what is needed. Your growing patience with yourself, even your self-compassion, is the fruit of being pursued, known, and loved by God.

After all, the same God who whispers, "Who told you?" and offers a "Peace be with you," dwells within, by the Spirit, joining his hello to yours.

RESOURCES

- Alison Cook and Kimberly Miller, *Boundaries for Your Soul: How to Turn Your Overwhelming Thoughts and Feelings into Your Greatest Allies*
- Ann Weiser Cornell, *The Power of Focusing: A Practical Guide to Emotional Self-Healing*
- Jenna Riemersma, *Altogether You: Experiencing Personal and Spiritual Transformation with Internal Family Systems Therapy*
- Elizabeth O'Connor, *Our Many Selves: A Handbook for Self-Discovery*

Reflection

1. Have you seen *Inside Out*? If not, take some time to watch it, perhaps with a friend or loved one. How does it help you personify parts of you that vie for control within you? Can you name your own inner characters? How does naming these parts of you elicit compassion for them?

2. What parts of you have you sometimes considered bad or unwanted? Examine one of them and see if you can't become curious about the role it has played within you. If you were to tell your story from the perspective of just

this one part of you, how would you tell it? If this goes well, try doing the same thing for more parts of you.

3. What is your first instinct when you experience an uncomfortable emotion or bodily sensation? Most of us want it to go away. Journal or talk to a friend about this instinct within you. See if you can find a concrete example. And then through the practices below, see if you might greet that emotion or sensation with a hello next time it arises. See if you might ask it what it's trying to tell you.

4. What is it like to consider that God sees you to the core and calls you "Beloved"? Who are people in your life who offer the kind "hello" of Jesus, who mirror your image-bearing worth, belonging, and purpose to you?

Practice: Say Hello

Practicing hello throughout your day

Spend a day focused on greeting whatever arises in you with a "hello" or even a "peace be with you." Whatever you sense arising within—sadness, a headache, an inner critic, anxiety— see if you might just turn toward it with some curiosity and kindness. See if you might greet that emotion or sensation the next time it arises and ask it what it's trying to tell you. We spend a lot of energy avoiding uneasy and uncomfortable inner experiences or emotions, so this exercise may feel unnatural or challenging. It's sometimes helpful to find a companion who might agree to do this with you for a day, and to compare notes about what shifted within you. At the end of the exercise, see if your inner experience is any different than it might've been the previous day. What feels different? What needs more attention and curiosity?

Get to know a part of you

Simply begin by noticing whatever emotion, thought, body sensation, or image is most present. Try to pay close attention to this as a distinct part of you. If possible, get a sense of where you experience this part of you in or around your body. See if you get an idea of what it looks like, how it relates to you, how old it is. Don't be surprised if you get a really clear image or inner experience of this part of you. How do you feel toward it? Can you find your way to compassion and curiosity for it? How does this part of you feel when you offer it compassion and curiosity? What does it want to share with you about how it feels? What it needs? What its experience has been? What role has this part played for you/in you? What would happen if it wasn't so extreme or if it softened a bit? What positive role could it play within you?

Acknowledge impact

When parts of us become extreme (what the ancient sages called "passions"), they can block us from joy, cut us off from our sense of clarity/agency/freedom, entrap us, alienate us from ourselves and others, and even manifest in harm to ourselves or others. In the Christian tradition, this is called *disorder* or *sin*. And it's helpful to get really clear about how this is happening within you so that you can be freed from its grip. So get to know one extreme part of yourself. It might be an inner critic, an angry part, an overeating part, a procrastinating part, a jealous part, a sad part. Practice the parts exercise on page 127. See if you can get some clarity around why it became so extreme. How was it trying to help you, and how did it end up hurting you or others? Can you empathize with it? And then, can you begin to become curious about or perhaps even acknowledge its painful impact on you or others? How does living from this more extreme part create more disorder and disconnection within you or in your relationships? And what might recognizing its impact through repentance (*metanoia*) look like?

Repentance often comes with a sense of grief for how living in that disordered way has caused ourselves and others pain, yet it's instrumental to the internal reordering we seek. Parts of us want to be free from their extreme roles, their fiery passions. Here, you might imagine Jesus greeting this part of you, not with anger but with delight, eager to know your heart, longing to see you live freely and fully. This isn't about self-contempt but about experiencing the compassionate embrace of the father in Luke 15.

HIDDEN ROOTS

Honoring What Is Known and Unknown
about Our Suffering

*Tell me what you fear and I will tell you what
has happened to you.*

D. W. WINNICOTT

IN THE EARLY MORNING HOURS of my fiftieth birthday, I quietly
gathered my journal, a favorite book, and a dry towel, tiptoe-
ing in the dark around our hotel room in Florida as Sara and
the girls slept. I was the first one to the beach that morning,
and I greeted the rising sun as a friend who'd been waiting for
someone to acknowledge his stunning glory. I walked the beach
gathering stones for a bit, all the while aware that I was avoiding
an inevitable conversation with myself.

I took a deep breath and acknowledged the unspoken ache
within. Truth be told, I felt scared, insecure, even unsure of
myself. Angry that I wasn't further along after years of my own

counseling, after hundreds of books consumed, after engaging in all manner of self-care practices. Ashamed that I, as a person who has written on wholeheartedness, still felt so scattered at times. Frustrated with myself that I so quickly reacted in anxiety and simmered with resentment. Sad that I'd gone it alone for so many years. I had imagined turning fifty as an inauguration into mature adulthood, into days of growing contentedness, eroding anxiety, burgeoning confidence, sage wisdom. A disgusted inner critic within whispered, *What is wrong with you? You ought to be much further along than you are. You'll never grow up.*

Behind me, a crew was setting up chaise lounges and umbrellas for beachgoers. I made my way over and handed the attendant a fifty-dollar bill for a setup for two, roiling within as I tallied the high cost of relaxation. I sat. And I couldn't do anything. My journal and book remained in my backpack. Here, on this day, I wasn't going to try to figure myself out. I couldn't. I just sat back, closed my eyes, and took a deep breath.

Inside, I could feel a surprising settling. And then a most unexpected voice:

I'm here, Chuck. You're not alone. You're loved. You're right where you need to be. And you're going to be okay.

I don't regularly have experiences of hearing from God, but I knew this voice was the kind whisper of the Spirit within me. Tears streamed as I let go of my self-judgments and received the care I needed.

Out of the Spotlight, into Surrender

Perhaps you, too, picked up this book hoping that this one—of all the many you've read—might provide that elusive clue to what's wrong with you. I get it. And I sincerely hope that what you're reading meets you right where you are and provides some frame for your experience. But in this chapter, I want to offer you a wider lens for your suffering, with the earnest hope that you'll be able to approach it with more gentleness, patience, humility, and empathy. That you'll recognize you're not a problem to be fixed, though your intentional work on yourself certainly matters.

Because here's what I've learned: Sometimes our holiest and most humbling encounters arise out of surrender. Of course, there are practices and resources—this book is filled with them!—that you can employ to intentionally engage with what's happening within and journey toward wholeness. But the truth remains that, even after all the work, the most profound moments of your transformation may occur when you've exhausted your resources.

While God's second question, "Who told you?" invites us to remember our stories, this work doesn't come with a guarantee of complete resolution of all that has ailed us. CJ, a client of mine who'd started counseling two years before, expressed frustration at how slow the work was going. "I just want to figure myself out!" he said.

"Your life isn't a math equation," I responded. "It's not a riddle to be solved." We spent the next couple of sessions exploring the pressure he'd felt to get fixed.

The late priest and poet John O'Donohue laments the ways in which we sometimes subject our stories to the glaring spotlight of anxious analysis, to an exhausting and unhelpful introspection:

> Negative introspection damages the soul. It holds many people trapped for years and years, and ironically, it never allows them to change. It is wise to allow the soul to carry on its secret work in the night side of your life. You might not see anything stirring for a long time. You might have only the slightest intimations of the secret growth that is happening within you, but these intimations are sufficient. We should be fulfilled and satisfied with them. You cannot dredge the depths of the soul with the meagre light of self-analysis. The inner world never reveals itself cheaply. Perhaps analysis is the wrong way to approach our inner dark.[1]

O'Donohue's words are a reminder that your soul doesn't respond well to coercion, confrontation, demands, fixing, rushing, tinkering, analyzing, and mastering. You were slow-cooked in your mother's womb; your body and soul formed to respond to presence, connection, safety, and attunement. Think about it. You're much more apt to connect and offer your vulnerability amidst soft candlelight and in conversation with a dear friend than under the bright lights of an interrogation room where you're being asked to solve a whodunit.

And yet, instead, we sometimes place our problems under

the stark lights of questioning and cross-examination. *What's wrong with me?* CJ asked himself. And so did I. We ask these questions of ourselves and perhaps of God, too, often with a sense of frustration and with a demand—I need to know, right now, what's wrong and how to fix it.

O'Donohue calls this mentality the "neon consciousness."[2]

You'll find this neon consciousness in some churches, where the glaring beams focus solely on your sinful behavior, your guilt and shame only magnified under the lights. You'll find it in therapeutic spaces where the goal is to shine the blazing lights of diagnosis in an attempt to analyze and conquer what ails you. You'll find it anywhere you are viewed more as a problem to be fixed than a person to be known.

In these spaces and places, your gut may tell you it's not safe, and it's wise to listen well to this inner wisdom. You may come to realize that your heart is too precious to be subjected to the harsh beams of interrogation. You don't stand accused. Nor are you a puzzle to be solved. Walk away if you ever experience this severe exposure. Because in the end, a neon consciousness fails to see that your soul is a vast expanse, a wild country, with wide open valleys and dark ocean depths. It fails to see that the wilderness journey within these 1,185 chapters unfolds slowly, requiring patience.

There are challenges we can see and name, to be sure, but there are mysteries too.

Sometimes without our practicing or prompting, our souls find their way to a deeper conversation we need to have, both within and with God. Here, we're mysteriously opened to a portal of grace that is precisely what we need in that moment. Here, we can relax and honor what we can't control, what we can't fix, even what we can't know about our stories and our sufferings. Here, we're invited to surrender.

God's compassionate questions in the Garden—and to our own souls—are invitations, not demands requiring immediate response, not inquiries demanding immediate answers. In fact, as we see in Genesis 3 and beyond, nothing was fixed quickly. Things only broke down further. Perhaps this, too, is to be expected, a mysterious unfolding that doesn't work on our timetables. And perhaps God's posture in Genesis 3 reveals a way of meeting one another that invites us to offer our*selves*, which is very different than offering our*solves*.

A Gentler Posture

A pivotal learning moment for me came in my work with a client named Kim. She was a late-twenty-something Black woman who'd seen multiple therapists for years. Kim struggled with chronic anxiety that manifested in night terrors, intrusive negative thoughts, and feelings of worthlessness. She would work tirelessly with each therapist, examining every angle of her life in order to understand the source of these deeply ingrained feelings. But for almost eight years, it remained a mystery.

When I first started seeing her, she sighed. "I'm not sure I want to start over again," she told me. "I just feel broken, unfixable, a problem no therapist can solve."

Week after week, we'd explore further. "I'm not sure we're

getting anywhere either," she said. My own anxiety grew as I wondered what I was missing.

So I turned up the neon lights.

The bright glare of analysis showed none of the typical signs that might lead to the rather significant symptoms of trauma she was experiencing. Her parents were exceptionally present and engaged. She was safe in the home she grew up in. She excelled in academics and athletics, particularly basketball. She had longtime, trusted friends. The longer we sat together, the more inadequate I felt; there was no smoking gun, nothing to make sense of her pain.

And so I gave up. I told her one day that I didn't have much more to ask or offer. She sighed, deep and relieved. "Thank goodness," she said. "This whole therapy thing has been exhausting."

We laughed. Honestly, it may have been the first time I felt truly relaxed and connected to her. "Well," I surmised, "we've looked for what went wrong, so now I'd love to know what went right. Bring in some of your high school photo albums next week and tell me some stories about the basketball championship." She was relaxed and even excited for our next session. That was a first for both of us.

And so in the weeks after, she shared stories. The neon lights were off now. She belly laughed with a freedom I'd not seen or heard from her before. She shed tears of gratitude and even grief as she reckoned with the passing of time since that championship year when she set the school record for points in a season. And those who knew Kim well could sense that something was shifting within her.

Eventually, we began to talk about when therapy might end. And it was exactly here, at what seemed to be the end, that a new beginning emerged.

Kim was seated on my couch with yet another photo album on her lap, sharing stories with me. On this particular day, she sat back, folding her legs under her on the couch and pulling a blanket over her lap. She smiled as she scanned a particular photo. And then she cocked her head, ever so slightly. It was an expression I'd never seen before.

"Where'd you go just now?" I asked. An echo of God's first question.

She was quiet, her eyes searching. This time, there'd be no bright lights of interrogation, no intrusive questions from me. Instead, we sat in silence together, simply honoring what was emerging.

When she was ready, she finally spoke. "It's funny, you know," she said. Again, she paused. She shook her head again, speechless, as if she'd finally stumbled onto an elusive clue. "It's just," she began again, "I'm the only Black face in all of those high school photographs."

With that, Kim closed her eyes and breathed deeply, exhaling and nodding her head as if affirming a truth she'd always known but never recognized. She wasn't devastated, but I could sense a hovering sadness. We sat longer. There was no rush.

"What's that say to you?" I responded. An echo of God's second question.

I sat as she shed tears. "The pain feels really deep, hundreds of years old inside of me," Kim said. Ten, even twenty minutes went by, Kim quietly weeping, both us aware of each other's tender presence, a connection we wouldn't spoil with words.

After some time, discerning that something deep had moved through her, she took a breath. "Thank you for being here and for honoring that grief," Kim said. In those sacred moments, I sensed that some mysterious alchemy was at work beyond our control, that this breakthrough of sorts couldn't have been manufactured. It was all a gift.

With Kim's help, I began to learn how to honor the mystery of our suffering.

It might be strange to hear this from someone like me. I'm a licensed therapist and an ordained pastor, and I train pastors and counselors to bring clarity and healing to those who are in need. But I admit that at least part of why I could write my last book, *When Narcissism Comes to Church*, is because I am familiar with the terrain. No, I'm not one for stage theatrics, and people don't experience me as grandiose or bullying. Yet, for too many years, I lived under the illusion that if I could just spend enough time with someone and if I could do a thorough enough survey of their past, I'd find the source of their pain and lead them to the healing they longed for. If that's not narcissistic, I'm not sure what is.

I'll let you in on a secret: Many of us suffer the great anxiety of not being able to help in ways we hoped we could. We're wearied when, despite our best efforts, a person's beleaguering symptoms continue on, or a marriage we thought we could save ends in a bitter divorce. (Who taught us it was our business to *save* in the first place?) Pastors seem to feel this acutely; they're burdened by the competition, the comparison, the compulsion to put the best product out there in order to survive. One pastor I counsel said, "I got into this to help people and left feeling hurt and helpless myself."

Too often we live with the expectation that a so-called expert might finally see what no one else has seen and offer the missing fix. Sometimes the better approach is to go easy with ourselves and others. Try softer, as my friend Aundi Kolber suggests.[3] Your soul isn't in a rush; it simply longs for the space to be known.

The Ancient Story Within

Working with Kim led me to greater curiosity about the ancestral and generational wounds people hold in their bodies. And it prompted me to wonder if God's "Who told you?" might invite us to reflect, not just on our own lives and stories, but also on those who came before us.

The waves of trauma that crash on your shores might not at all be connected to what happened to *you*, but rather distant echoes of ancestral pain whose source you may only catch a glimpse of on the horizon. Resmaa Menakem's wise and prophetic work *My Grandmother's Hands* offers the humbling reminder that you bear the stories of your parents and grandparents, even your distant ancestors, in your body. That pain can be hidden in your genes and transmitted epigenetically from generation to generation, expressed at any time, through any number of triggers.[4]

Of course, this mysterious phenomenon is true for all of us, but Menakem describes the agonizing experience of many people of color, writing

The answer to why so many of us have difficulties is because our ancestors spent centuries here under unrelentingly brutal conditions. Generation after generation, our bodies stored trauma and intense survival energy, and passed these on to our children and grandchildren.[5]

In the months after her revelation, Kim's symptoms lifted. More importantly, her image-bearing inheritance of worth, belonging, and purpose was claimed with new freedom and joy. She even grew in a sense of solidarity with her ancestors, amidst unanswered questions and untold stories. "I don't have to have it all figured out," she said. "I can be open to days of gladness and other days of grief. My body will let me know."

God's "Who told you?" offers us, like Kim, the opportunity to honor the unknown, to acknowledge the stories that we may not know or may never know, to recognize the pain in our bodies that spans generations. It can be painful, even heartbreaking, to honor that which is seemingly unknown or unresolvable. And for this reason, we must be gentle with one another, for everyone you meet is fighting a great battle, a battle caught up in a much larger story.

The unseen suffering requires gentle tending. Our rush to fix that which is visible may cause us to ignore that which lies beneath it, that which doesn't reveal itself cheaply. Just the other day, I overheard a chat at a local coffee shop between two women who seemed to be friends, both in their early- to midthirties, one offering the other a window into her marital issues. With each new disclosure, the friend would interject—"Have you tried this?" or "Have you read that?" The neon lights were bright, and I was exhausted just listening. It was not a soul-honoring exchange.

In contrast to this anxious posture aimed at targeting, analyzing, and fixing, we can choose to be with and bear witness. We can trust that what needs to be seen and spoken will reveal itself in the safety of presence and connection. We can trust that what needs to be processed will, indeed, be processed in good time. After all, God shows up, not to fix, but with presence and compassion, offering questions bathed in curiosity.

Awakening to Our Primal Wound

God's story for us began in beautiful intimacy and goodness, but Adam and Eve soon found themselves east of Eden. Our stories begin in unfathomable intimacy, but whispers of a rupture arrive before we're ready. Too early in life, our "eyes are opened" (see Genesis 3:7), just as Adam and Eve's were—to pain, to sadness, to separation, to shame, sometimes even to death. We awaken to the reality that the waves of their ancient trauma reach our shores, alerting us to a primal wound within, which echoes their original ache.

I first heard "primal wound" in a talk by a Franciscan priest, but later I learned that some account of this wound is told across most religions. Suffering, and its roots in disconnection, has long been mused on by philosophers, poets, mystics, theologians, and psychologists. Psychotherapists John Firman and Ann Gila write

> [The primal wound is] a break in the intricate web
> of relationships in which we live, move, and have
> our being. A fundamental trust and connection to
> the universe is betrayed, and we become strangers
> to ourselves and others, struggling for survival in a
> seemingly alien world. In psychological terms, our
> connection to our deeper Self is wounded. In religious
> and philosophical terms, it is our connection to
> Ultimate Reality, the Ground of Being, or the Divine
> that is broken. No matter how we elect to describe it,
> the fact remains that this wounding cuts us off from
> the deeper roots of our existence.[6]

In the Christian tradition, Genesis 3 offers an ancient story of our suffering, sin, even sabotage. In it, we see echoes of our doubt and shame, our anxiety and self-protection. Adam and Eve doubted, and we doubt too. Adam and Eve grasped, and so do we. Adam and Eve hid, and we hide in countless ways. And each of us is invited to explore how the ancient disconnection arrives on our personal shores, how we experience it within, how it manifests in inexplicable heartache, unrelenting longing, and disordered ways of loving. All echoes of the primal wound.

My own eyes were opened when I was just seven or eight years old. It was stunning and severe, a sure sign that I'd traversed east of Eden.

Our family had been retreating with our church in a heavenly setting at the Delaware Water Gap, enjoying long, sunshine-filled summer days of laughter and limitless lemonade. We would retire in the evenings to the safety of our Volkswagen camper, our beloved home away from home on wheels. It felt to me like the very center of the Garden of Eden. My bed was elevated above in the pop-top, and I'd gaze up into the deep black sky, counting the stars until my eyes became too heavy.

On a perfect afternoon, we launched tubes into a slow, rolling river, my tube maybe a hundred yards behind my best friend from church. With my parents and some friends, I meandered slowly, losing track of time as we splashed and snickered all the way, beautifully surrendered to the flowing waters. This was perfection.

I hadn't quite noticed that we'd lost sight of my friend until I saw the commotion farther down the river. People seemed panicked. Immediately, I sensed my parents' anguish and confusion. We exited the river in silence, navigating our way back to camp.

I later learned that my best friend had been sucked into a whirlpool that no one noticed, drowning before his parents could save him.

Genesis 3:7 says "their eyes were opened" (NLT), and my eyes were opened that day, to terror, to overwhelm, to bewilderment, to death.[7] My parents recognized my confusion and sadness, and that probably saved me from the traumatic overwhelm of the moment. But even the comfort of my parents could not reach the place within me that felt desperately alone, anguished, and inconsolable.

That primal wound had awakened within me, arriving on my shores, my body remembering the ancient breach Adam and Eve experienced. An aching loneliness had entered into my childhood Eden.

My friend's death didn't cause it. But it did awaken me to a more primal ache, a pivotal moment in which I first began to sense life's fragility. It's as if the serpent was whispering in my ear, "You see, the world isn't safe. God can't be trusted. Pain is right around the corner." It's an ache that runs deeper than the things that happened to us, an ache revealed as an ancient story that lives on within us. This wound, among all others, sits at the subterranean core of our being, the hidden root of our suffering. Psychologist and former Trappist monk James Finley writes,

> On the one hand there is the great truth that from the first moment of my existence the deepest dimension of my life is that I am made by God for union with himself. The deepest dimension of my identity as a human person is that I share in God's own life both now and in eternity in a relationship of untold intimacy.
>
> On the other hand, my own daily experience impresses upon me the painful truth that my heart has listened to the serpent instead of to God.

There is something in me that puts on fig leaves
of concealment, kills my brother, builds towers of
confusion, and brings cosmic chaos upon the earth.
There is something in me that loves darkness rather
than light, that rejects God and thereby rejects my own
deepest reality as a human person made in the image
and likeness of God.[8]

Both stories, true at the same time. Both realities—
connection and disconnection—live on within us. We bear the
wounds of what happened to us. We bear ancestral wounds,
passed on through generations. We bear a primal wound, an
intuition in our deep memory of Eden and how we've been
severed from it. There aren't neon lights bright enough to make
sense of it all.

And yet, God, the Compassionate Witness, comes near.
Jesus, God in the flesh, joins in suffering solidarity with us.
The Spirit bears witness within us. We are not alone in any of it.

The Practice of Blessing What Is Known and Unknown

We can honor the hidden roots of our sufferings, the mystery
that is us. To be sure, this does not mean that we ignore the
inner work—the exploration of our stories, our attachment patterns, even our many selves. But there are seasons to lean in
to what is known and can be healed, and there are seasons to
embrace the darkness, to acknowledge the immensity of one's
story, the vastness of the soul, the mystery of the unknown.

It doesn't always provide the clarity or the closure we long for. Such was the case for Wendy, a friend who began counseling with a capable therapist in the late 2000s after she identified the narcissistic emotional and sexual abuse she had endured from the senior pastor she had worked for. She took her abuse seriously, working hard to tease out the confusing gaslighting she encountered—and, eventually, recognizing that none of it was her fault. She sought justice in a church trial for her senior pastor and triumphed; other victims were identified, and the senior pastor was forced to leave ministry. I and all of her friends were so proud of her, for her inner work, for her courage, for her perseverance.

Years after this reckoning, we sat together over coffee, reflecting on what that season of her life had taught her. For a long time, she mused, she was fueled by the idea that justice would grant her needed relief from the trauma of it all. "Someone needed to pay," she said, "or so I thought."

And while it helped a bit, it didn't magically heal the traumatic wounds the pastor had left behind. "It helped to know he couldn't hurt anyone else," Wendy told me, "but I was still hurting." She then embarked on what she would come to call her "eight-year therapeutic odyssey," a season where she worked vigorously to understand herself and her story more clearly.

Sitting in the coffee shop, listening to her recount these difficult years, I could sense her face softening as she shared vulnerable details about learning to forgive those who hurt her. Her voice fell just above a whisper. "I even had to forgive God for not being the quick-acting police officer responding on cue to my frequent 911 prayers," Wendy admitted. "I had to let a lot of what I believed about God die so that I could rediscover goodness and mercy. All shall be well."

Sitting with her, I could feel the goodness and mercy she spoke of. She embodied it. But knowing the vulnerable details of her story, I never would've expected her to quote the medieval English Christian mystic Julian of Norwich.[9] "How did you get from 'someone needs to pay' to 'all shall be well'?" I asked, curious.

I peered intensely into her gentle and wise eyes, really wanting to know, even for myself. A part of me wondered briefly if she, like many, was simply bypassing her pain spiritually, enlisting hollow, clichéd phrases to distance themselves from the reality of the harm that had been done to them. Yet, I also knew that Wendy had done the work. Her "all shall be well" had to have been born out of suffering, not claimed as an excuse to avoid it.

She smiled. "I simply knew that a time had come for me to honor the mystery of my story—what I've discovered and what will remain undiscovered—and walk more gently into my next season of life," she said quietly. With that, she sipped her last bit of tea. I sat back in wonder. I texted a friend: "I just met a real-life grown-up."

May we all find a little bit of Wendy in our own stories. All shall be well, even if it takes a little longer than we had hoped.

RESOURCES

- James Finley, *The Healing Path: A Memoir and an Invitation*
- Resmaa Menakem, *My Grandmother's Hands: Racialized Trauma and the Pathway to Mending Our Hearts and Bodies*
- John O'Donohue, *Anam Ċara: A Book of Celtic Wisdom*
- Mark Wolynn, *It Didn't Start with You: How Inherited Family Trauma Shapes Who We Are and How to End the Cycle*

Reflection

1. Have you experienced moments when the books, podcasts, or other resources you've engaged with just don't seem to help, and when you've felt a sense of powerlessness or wondered how you'll get the help and care you need? How does this sense of powerlessness feel? When this happens, are you apt to redouble your efforts? Or descend into frustrated resignation? How could you try to approach this sense of powerlessness as a gift to be welcomed?

2. As you reflect on the "neon consciousness" that sometimes shows up in church, therapy, or other spaces, when/where/with whom have you known the pressure of demand, analysis, fixing, tinkering, controlling, and more? How did you respond? What approach would you have preferred?

3. Consider the mystery of your own unfolding story and the trauma you bear in your body, some of which is wrapped up in your ancestral story and some of which is an ancient and shared story of humanity's disconnection. How does that perspective help you approach your own inner work with more patience, gentleness, and grace? How might you open yourself to this larger frame for holding your own story?

Practice: Blessing What Is Known and Unknown

The three candles

To begin this practice, find a quiet place where you can light three candles. Each represents a different aspect of engaging your life and story.

- The first candle represents what is known in your story. Light this candle to honor what you've learned about yourself. Perhaps you've been on your own journey in therapy or seeking spiritual direction, or maybe you've sat with a friend or a pastor where together you've named places of pain, possibly even patterns of self-sabotage or addiction. Allow a few moments to breathe and honor this good, good work. Offer gratitude to the different parts of yourself you've gotten to know along the way. Listen for the whisper of the Spirit within saying, "Well done."

148

- The second candle represents what is yet to be discovered as you continue your work. In the days and weeks to come, you may peel back yet another layer of your story. Light this candle to honor your ongoing desire to live in truth, your desire for God to search you and know your heart (Psalm 139:23-24). Honor the challenges of this work. Honor the many resources it requires. Honor your persistence. Honor the parts of you that sometimes feel like it's too much. Honor your surrender to the unpredictable timetable of the work. Honor your deep longing to be well.

- The third candle represents what is unknown and perhaps at some level even unknowable. Light this candle to honor what you may never know, understand, or resolve. Light it not as an act of passivity or even complicity, but as a surrendering to what you can't control. Remember that even the saints in heaven awaiting the second coming of Jesus cry out "How long?" (Revelation 6:10). Honor the depths of your own cry of "How long, O Lord?" Honor the feelings that come up here, whether you find fear, sadness, or even rage. You may wrestle with this if you feel a great need to figure out what happened or desperately want a wrong to be righted or an abuser to be held accountable. If needed, honor your hesitancy to light this candle and wait until you feel ready.

PART 3

HAVE YOU

Seeking the Source of Our Hunger,

EATEN

Navigating the Mystery,

FROM THE

and Learning to Long for So Much More

TREE?

ADDICTION AND GRACE

Where We Take Our Hunger

The story of Eden is not over, yet neither is it simply repeating
itself endlessly through history. Instead, it is going somewhere.
I believe that humankind's ongoing struggle with addiction
is preparing the ground of perfect love.

GERALD G. MAY

SUE WANDERS INTO MY church counseling center office in tears, emotionally bruised and beaten. She's been caught in marital infidelity and shamed by friends and church leaders. The prospect of losing her marriage and children looms large. She despises what she's done and, even more, the craving to keep doing it.

She sits across from me, barely able to raise her eyes.

"Can you look at me?" I ask. She struggles to make eye contact, deep in shame.

"Can I ask you a different kind of question than the one everyone else has asked?" I said. "What were you longing for?"

The Lure of the Lie Within

"Have you eaten from the tree?"

Years ago, when I first began reflecting on the questions posed by God in Genesis 3, I struggled to hear kindness in this third question. It felt too obviously ridden with accusation and disappointment, an angry Father determined to hear the worst confirmed. But in time, I began to sense a deep grief—a Father who'd offered everything to Adam and Eve only to see them, like Edmund in *The Lion, the Witch and the Wardrobe*, throw it all away for some Turkish delight.

We're not told, but I sometimes wonder how long Adam and Eve waited to eat from the tree, pondering their predicament. Scripture says, "When the woman saw that the fruit of the tree was good for food and pleasing to the eye, and also desirable for gaining wisdom, she took some and ate it" (Genesis 3:6). But how long did it take to get to Eve's "when"? Did she and Adam sleep on it? Did they experience a growing emptiness that caused their bellies to ache? Did the fruit look better and better as they grew hungrier and hungrier for it? How long before they decided that the forbidden fruit could tamp the ache and offer them the fullness they sought, and perhaps even more?

How long does it take you and me?

Each of us is born into a world where the possibility of goodness, fullness, and flourishing awaits, where our image-bearing sense of worth, belonging, and purpose might be uniquely discovered and embodied as we grow and mature. We're born with indispensable needs to feel safe, seen, soothed, and secure.

But soon enough we, too, will hear the lie of disconnection.

We'll hear echoes of that ancient serpent's whisper, voices that contradict God's pronouncement of our inherent beloved-ness. The ancient intruder in Genesis plants the lie that our image-bearing worth, belonging, and purpose can't be trusted, that God's goodness can't be counted on. That if we're going to make it, we'll have to make it on our own. And until God makes all things new (Revelation 21:5), we'll continue to experience the ache of incompleteness, even an insatiable hunger for fullness.

To be sure, at our best we'll seek to meet our needs in healthy ways and through good and secure connections, with God and with others. But more often, grasping for more from the in-between in which we live, we discover the magic elixir of self-soothing. "I've learned a thousand ways to cope," a retreat participant once told me, "and they're all easier than healing." These words sting with honesty. *That's the lie*, I thought to myself when I heard them. That's the root of the ancient fallacy, one we've acted on for time immemorial. We've fallen for the lie that a bit of drink here and an hour of scrolling there will quell the deep ache of our hearts, the lie that keeps us from attending to what's happening within, where our wounds fester.

But it's here, in our spaces of self-soothing and our places of pain management, that God once again meets us.

"Have you eaten from the tree?" he asks, which is to say, "Where have you taken your hunger?" His tone is not one of rageful anger but of somber curiosity: "Talk to me about the ways you've been suffering alone, coping on your own. Tell me where you've gone to quell the ache." Somehow, in this third question, God invites Adam and Eve—and us—to wonder about what we've wrapped our hearts around, what we've become addicted to in our attempts to self-medicate. Still present, still listening, still compassionate, he meets us in our exposed shame; he moves toward us with tenderness and invites us to be healed, not through self-soothing but through love, not by willpower but by grace.

The Problem *of* Addiction?

"Addictions at their root are about disconnection and the managing of pain from that disconnection," writes a dear friend and veteran therapist Dawn Elliott Kendall.[1] Our own addictions may show up in a myriad of ways, through food and drink, in sex and scrolling, in controlling and codependency. Amidst Storms that stir within, we may choose something that numbs our ache or dulls our anxiety. Amidst the Fog that envelops, we may seek self-harm or substance abuse. But regardless of what we choose, our addictions are always seen as a potential solution to disconnection, an attempt to soothe our dysregulated bodies and find relief on our own terms.

None of us are immune. Even the most securely attached and well-loved among us experience the sting of loss, rejection, misunderstanding, disappointment, and failure. "I cried when I was born and every day shows why," wrote the seventeenth-century poet and priest George Herbert.[2] If each of us bears the wound of traumatic disconnection this side of heaven, then each of us is bound to self-soothe in addiction. It's an equal playing field; we can't split the world into the wounded and the well, the addict and the abstinent.

This reality humbles us, and most often we learn the hard way. During my first clinical internship, I was assigned to a men's addiction group. As we greeted one another at the opening session, I announced to the men that I was simply a facilitator (not an addict like them).

Then they started sharing their stories. As they named their ways of coping and described the binds they experienced, I was proven wrong time and time again. I walked out the front door with them in tears. I was one of them. Of course I was.

Around that time, I found my way to Gerald G. May's *Addiction and Grace*, a book of immense beauty and wisdom written by a man kind enough to engage me in some long-distance spiritual direction over the next year. Under May's tutelage, I learned that my heart was more cluttered with attachments than I'd imagined, my hands grasping for whatever breadcrumb I could find to satiate my hunger. A host of addictions came to light, not least my most precious ones as a cavalier seminary student: certainty and self-righteousness.

But I also learned that there was grace in the light. Instead of seeing these addictions as problems to be solved, we began to uncover the deeper ache and anxiety beneath my behaviors. This proved to be a wonderfully gracious perspective, one too few operate from. Often, the focus of addiction recovery goes one of two ways: either it emphasizes the problem of moral failure rooted in individuals' fallen nature, requiring them to accept their identity as sinners and to turn from their sin to lives of abstinence and obedience; or it underscores the problem of flawed biology and an inherited condition, requiring individuals to accept their identity as addicts by abstaining and seeking sobriety and accountability among fellow addicts. Both paths treat the addiction *as* the problem rather than seeing it as *an attempt to solve* a deeper problem. And both, perhaps unwittingly, leave one with the feeling that there's something deeply wrong with them at the core of their being.

Indeed, the truth of addiction is that it is embedded in a larger story. It can't be reduced to depravity or disease, behavior or biology. Biography holds the key. Consider the words of the early twentieth-century English poet D. H. Lawrence:

> *I am ill because of wounds to the soul, to the deep*
> >   *emotional self*
> *and the wounds to the soul take a long, long time, only time*
> >   *can help*
> *and patience, and a certain difficult repentance.*[3]

Our underlying wounds need attending to. We've got to ask ourselves: What role does addiction play in our story? How is it an attempt to address our deep hunger, our unquenchable thirst, our aching emptiness, our lingering loneliness, our debilitating dysregulation, our traumatizing sense of disconnection? How is it an attempt to reconstruct a sense of worth, belonging, and purpose in a way that ultimately sabotages each?

When we begin to think this way, we see that addiction isn't the problem; it's the attempted solution to the perplexing pain underneath it.

Addiction as a Signpost

"What were you longing for?" I ask Sue that day in my office, an echo of God's third question. Her pain and guilt over her infidelity palpable, she says, sobbing, "I've longed to be seen and valued in the way he saw and valued me." Tears stream down her face.

"Of course," I say. "Who wouldn't want that?"

She looks up incredulously. She expected condemnation, not kindness. But doesn't God meet Adam and Eve in their crushing shame and self-made remedies? He doesn't turn his back—he turns his gracious face toward them—and his curiosity and compassion are compelling. Indeed, this safe kindness is what opens the door to true understanding: Beyond Sue's behavior is biography, a story of a soul empty and alone in a challenging marriage; the story of a woman who, wounded by her father's absence in her childhood, had long ago found a working salve in the attention of boys. In the ache of disconnection, a part of us hungers for the temporary reprieve of some pseudo-connection.

It doesn't negate the wreckage. If Genesis 3 is any indication, addiction still comes with a cost. Adam and Eve will walk in the wilderness in the days to come, in a land of thorns and thistles, bearing the pain in their bodies, experiencing the rupture in their relationships. In the same way, we can't ignore the harmful debris field that often accompanies addiction—the broken trust, the severed relationships, the disruptions that extend to almost every area of life.

Biography never excuses harmful behavior, but it certainly invites us to attend to the wound out of which it occurs. "It is impossible to understand addiction," Gabor Maté writes, "without asking what relief the addict finds, or hopes to find, in the drug or the addictive behavior."[4] If trauma is not what happened to you but what happens within you, then you eventually need to turn your gaze to the wound.

And our addictions are signposts; they always point the way to the traumatic wound.

Self-Medicating our Disconnection

Trey wasn't buying what I was selling about the connection between trauma and addiction. He was a porn addict, and he just wanted to stop. He'd tried web-based accountability programs and 12-step groups. He'd attended healing prayer services. But after brief reprieves, he'd be back online, in an escalating addiction that was threatening his marriage and job.

"I'm not looking for some smoking gun from your past that will tell us why you struggle with this addiction," I told him as we sat together one day. I could tell he was getting frustrated with the process of therapy, how long it was taking to heal. "I'm simply curious about the story your addicted part wants to tell."

"My addicted part?" he asked, a bit confused by my language.

"I assume you aren't always in your addiction," I clarified. "I know there are parts of you that are self-giving in your marriage, faithful in your work, and even likely to make really healthy choices. But then it seems that, on occasion, your addicted part jumps in and takes the lead."

Trey was stunned. "I've always thought this was the core of me, but you're right," he said. "It's like he does just jump in and take me over at times."

This small separation made a big difference. Consumed by his shame, Trey had long believed this was the dark underbelly and deepest core of his being; but now, we focused in on this part of him—his thoughts and feelings when he felt in this addicted state, his appearance and even his age. With compassion and curiosity, we discovered that though Trey felt well-loved by his parents, he had experienced the ordinary challenges of childhood in a way that led him to internalize a sense of being excluded and unwanted. It wasn't a surprise that he felt about twelve years old in his addicted state. He was medicating a wound of disconnection that had started in the hallways and playground of his childhood school, a wound that left him with a burden of shame, soothed for a time with continued dopamine hits of porn.

What Trey's heart really longed for was belonging.

Trey wasn't addicted to sex. He was addicted to the soothing chemical cocktail an hour of pornography and masturbation would produce. And those neurochemical hits soothed the sting of shame and the ache of alienation. But as any addict knows, the craving only grows, the relief diminishes, and the short-term solution often leads to longer-term disconnection. The word *addiction* comes from the Latin *addicere*, which indicates being bound, even enslaved to something.

The very thing meant to free you ends up binding you.

In his provocative TED Talk, author Johann Hari says the opposite of addiction is not sobriety but connection.[5] Trey would eventually heal in reconnection, with himself, with God, and with a wife and good friends who saw the depths of who he was and who invited him to live more vulnerably and honestly before them. The addicted part of him that used to take over didn't need to take over anymore. The power of his addiction began to wane. Trey didn't need to chase something that was already his, in union and communion with God.

The Futility of the Chase

We know that so-called neural marketers target our cravings, and they capitalize, quite literally, on our restlessness. The research division at a top American auto manufacturer ponders "the organized creation of dissatisfaction," hoping a well-played advertisement for a luxury pickup truck might stir within you just enough unrest with the now outdated car you bought three years ago.[6] And how often do you, like me, notice that the grill you were telling your wife you needed mysteriously shows up in your Facebook feed?

It's the oldest trick in the book. The serpent slithers up alongside Adam and Eve whispering the lie that they're not enough, that they're missing something core, that God is holding out on them. We've been given everything we need, but the deceitful whisper sells us the lie that we've got to find it outside ourselves. Whether the lie comes from the serpent or a marketer, we are invited to chase: Chase love. Chase soothing. Chase acceptance. Chase achievement. Chase recognition. Chase numbness. Chase certainty. Chase perfection. I even have a little plastic card in my wallet with the words "Chase Freedom." The reality is, it's not a one-off addiction that we're dealing with; it's a whole way of living. We are immersed in an exhausting chase after those basic needs to feel safe, seen, soothed, and secure. The lie is that it's out there, the fruit on a tree, the bonus in your checking account, the seductive glance of the person sitting across from you in the coffee shop, the adrenaline hit of a well-timed truth bomb on social media. So we'll keep chasing, keep grasping, keep striving, even if it costs us in body and soul.

"Addiction begins as an attempt to induce feelings that we were biologically programmed to generate innately, and would have—if unhealthy development hadn't got in the way," writes Gabor Maté.[7] Maté's point: There is a core of goodness and delight within every newborn waiting to burst forth. And yet each of us is also born into a world of shattered shalom, where the serpent's sly lies eventually penetrate. In time, we begin to live from a story of deficiency. None of us are immune.

Consider the son who stayed home in Luke 15, the supposed good son who didn't run off with his father's inheritance like his prodigal brother. Even still, he seethed with jealousy and rage as his younger brother was welcomed home with gifts and a party. His addictions might not have mirrored his brother's, but he, too, was living in a story of deficiency, disconnected from his core of goodness and delight. He had forgotten about his irrevocable inheritance. We're not given the details of how, but clearly he'd been lulled into the chase too. But his compassionate father's words pointed him back to what is core. "'My son,' the father said, 'you are always with me, and everything I have is yours'" (Luke 15:31).

We chase after what is already ours. The sixteenth-century Spanish saint and reformer, Teresa of Ávila, understood this well. And she discovered an extraordinary metaphor for the chase. Old Roman aqueducts dotted the Spanish landscape of her day, with their extensive bridgework and large conduits testifying to once majestic and ingenious edifices. But now they sat abandoned, crumbling, useless. The construction of Roman aqueducts had required a massive effort, all to get desperately needed water. In them, she saw before her eyes your life and mine—the lives we build chasing it all—lives built on the lie that we've got to fill our own tanks. In them, she saw our eager striving, our massive efforts to get our needs met on our own. In them, she found a valuable lesson. The living water is already within, "bubbling forth," she writes. We don't need to engineer it, strive for it, chase after it. It's within, the living water of God. Stop chasing after it, she tells us. "We accomplish nothing by tiring ourselves"[8] in the process. Rather than medicating our sense of disconnection and deficiency, we can rest in our inheritance of worth, belonging, and purpose.

The Practice of Reading Signposts

In chapter 5, I invited you into the practice of saying hello. This exercise in self-compassion opens you to a conversation with hidden parts of yourself, a practice that can lead to profound healing. The movie *Inside Out* offered a compelling picture of our disordered emotions and a helpful hint at what it takes to start a conversation with the parts of ourselves that seem to take over at times.

In a similar way, seeing an addiction as a signpost invites us to greet it, too, with compassion and curiosity. Whether the addiction is to self-harming behavior, bingeing and purging, pornography, substances, gambling, gaming, control, certainty, a relationship, or a toxic religious belief system of some kind, when we become aware of the behavior and the harm it causes, we often want to be free of it.

In Christian contexts, we may become obsessed with behavioral change and mired in a moralism that may offer surface-level shifts but that sabotages deep healing. In an attempt to live faithfully, some of us go to great lengths and spend significant time trying self-help strategies, only to become further frustrated when they don't work. This is because addiction itself isn't the problem, but the sign and symptom of a more significant wound. If we don't treat the wound, we're likely to bounce between behavioral interventions that don't ultimately help.

Trey, for instance, had experienced the futility of repeated self-help, behavior-modification remedies. And so we took a new path together. He learned that when he greeted his addictive behavior, he was no longer demonizing it, but in a strange sense, dignifying it as his current (and maybe only!) means of coping, adapting, and surviving.

At first, Trey sensed that this part of him was dark, greedy, and "Gollum-like," a reference to a character in Tolkien's *The Lord of the Rings*. Gollum was a hobbit who'd become deformed and twisted in his covetous search to possess the ring of power. We wondered how showing curiosity and hospitality toward this Gollum-like part of him would change Trey's perspective. Trey closed his eyes, exhaling and opening himself to deeper contact. After a few moments of quiet, he said, "It's like I'm sensing that this really hungry part of me went searching for something empowering, something to fill him and finally let him be accepted."

His eyes showed their first sign of a tear since we'd started meeting. "He's tired."

"Of course he is," I validated. "And when you quelled that hunger, what kind of relief did it provide? What did it keep you from feeling?"

He closed his eyes again. "For about ten minutes, I wasn't lost, I wasn't a loser, I didn't feel like a reject. I felt strong and seen and satisfied." As he said this, the tears streamed more fully and freely. "And that's it. I'm still so scared of being rejected, of not being loved. Chuck, I don't even trust that my wife wants me."

His body began trembling, and he sobbed. I walked over and sat next to him on the couch, my hand on his back just below his shoulders, gently rubbing circles. "Shh," I whispered, knowing that the little boy within him needed soothing.

Once his weeping stopped, Trey spoke. He sounded defiant now, resolute. "I don't want a cheap chemical high. . . . I want love, real love."

It wasn't easy, but Trey followed the signpost to the wound: rejection, exclusion, the feeling of being unwanted, unseen. And with courage, he found an even deeper well: a well of longing, where he discovered a desire to be seen, accepted, loved. And of course, Trey's journey wasn't over. His wife was, understandably, hurt by the depth and deceit of his addiction, and it would take time for her to trust again. But instead of seeing this work as Trey's alone, she, too, became curious. In time, she'd begin to name a host of her own addictive tendencies, places where she'd experienced a neurochemical taste of Eden, only to find herself ashamed and alone. Though their behaviors were different, Trey and his wife awakened to how similar they were. And she, too, recognized that she'd been medicating a wound. Her courage to explore what was happening within her opened her to empathy for Trey, and together they began their wilderness journey back to themselves and one another.

I won't lie: This movement takes courage and patience. Trey and his wife's journey didn't end in an aha moment. In my work, there are too few Disney endings and many, many dark nights that people face as they seek further healing and transformation. Now in my midfifties and with decades of self-exploration behind me, I realize that what seem like mountaintop experiences fit for storybook endings are merely thresholds into deeper transformation. Saul's Damascus Road experience led to three years of soul-searching in the desert before he became Paul. Jonah's transformation required three days in the belly of the whale. Ruth faced a long, lonely road filled with loss. And Jesus endured the Cross.

The deepest work often happens when the lights go out.

RESOURCES

- Seth Haines, *The Book of Waking Up: Experiencing the Divine Love That Reorders a Life*
- Gabor Maté, *In the Realm of Hungry Ghosts: Close Encounters with Addiction*
- Gerald G. May, *Addiction and Grace: Love and Spirituality in the Healing of Addictions*

Reflection

1. How have you typically understood addiction? And how does it strike you to consider addiction not as a problem to be solved but as an attempt to solve a deeper problem? How might that shift your perspective on yourself or others in your life?

2. If we're all navigating some kind of trauma and if we're all attempting to comfort ourselves in some way, then each of us is invited to consider our everyday ways of self-soothing. Reflect on one or two common behaviors

you engage in that most might not see as addictive, but that represent a form of soothing (i.e., scrolling on your phone, spending hours playing video games or binge-watching shows, shopping). Consider what role this activity plays in your life. Is it something that is used to numb, distract, soothe, or stimulate?

3. If addiction isn't core to you or to anyone, if instead it's just an adaptation, a way of coping, even just a part of your trying to self-soothe, then imagine God meeting you for a conversation about one of your particular strategies for self-soothing. Take a few minutes to hear the question beneath the question God asks in Genesis 3 ("Where have you taken your hunger?") and sense the kindness of God's inquiry, the compassion in his voice. How does it feel to imagine God approaching you with compassion and kind-ness instead of condemnation for your bad behavior?

Practice: Reading the Signposts

Signpost awareness

Our addictions disconnect us, so an antidote of sorts is to bring attention and awareness to what you're doing in the moment you're doing it. This takes some intentionality and courage. And you'll likely notice some inner resistance. To practice this, you'll need to "catch yourself" in the act of self-soothing. So, for example, maybe you notice a pattern of scrolling and shop-ping online, not because you need those items but because it soothes and distracts. Follow the steps below, engaging them as nonjudgmentally as you can:

- First, speak out loud (if you're able) exactly what you're doing. Say, "I am scrolling and shopping online." Or "I'm pouring another glass of wine."
- Second, identify the feeling you might be escaping and the replacement feeling this activity offers. Perhaps you might say, "I was feeling empty and sad, and this helped me feel excited and full." Or "I was feeling rejected and alone, and this helped me feel connected and alive."
- Third, reflect on the deeper need this action is attempting to address. You can view this through the perspective of a hunger/thirst/longing for something you've been missing, or through the perspective of an ache or wound within that you're trying to medicate. Here are some examples:
  - "I think I'm longing for some sense of being seen and connected, and looking at porn offers me something of this."
  - "I think I have a need for some relief from the anxiety that buzzes in me, and a few drinks at night offer that needed relief."
- Finally, if you're able, bring some conscious choice to what happens next. Even if your choice is to continue, do it mindfully, aware of the feeling and the need.

When you have some distance from this episode, reconsider these same questions. But end by asking yourself if you want to continue to engage in this same pattern given what you know now. Perhaps you might ask yourself, *Is there a different path I can take next time?*

Getting to know the more frightening, addictive parts of yourself

Some of us are mindful of behaviors we'd be ashamed to name out loud. We may engage in self-harm by cutting, bingeing and purging, or taking illegal substances. We may be dealing with a chronic and long-term cycle of pornography and masturbation. We may be hiding how much we eat or drink. We may be secretly losing money in stock market trading that our spouse doesn't know about. Regardless, these actions often elicit much more shame and provoke more elaborate strategies to hide and cover up the behavior.

In such situations, it's often important to find a curious and compassionate, trauma-informed therapist to open up to. In fact, these more extreme behaviors are also parts of us that soothe, numb, distract, and self-medicate, and they won't respond to behavior modification or guilt-and-shame strategies for curbing the thoughts or behaviors. These parts of you are trying to get your inner needs met, albeit in ways that hurt you. They'll relent and relax, however, in a place of presence and in a space of safety. They'll abate as you seek to get your very real needs met in much healthier ways. This all begins with a radical honesty with yourself and a commitment to name what lurks in the shadows. See if you can engage the "signpost awareness" exercise on pages 169–171 with these more extreme parts of you, even in the moment. The more you can bring a compassionate presence to these moments and these parts of you, the more you'll see their power diminish.

THE DARK NIGHT

Healing What's Hidden in the Shadows

Christ of the mysteries, I trust You
to be stronger than each storm within me.
I will trust in the darkness and know
that my times, even now, are in Your hand.

ST. BRENDAN THE NAVIGATOR

ONE THURSDAY AFTERNOON, I sat in a familiar section of a Borders bookstore, cloistered away in a low-traffic nook between the feminist studies and the literature sections. It had become my regular practice over the years to spend all day Thursday in this space. I sat at the same table every time, writing sermons, preparing and praying, and connecting deeply with good friends. It was also at this table that I often encountered Jesus, a liminal time of visceral nearness; I felt him across from me, smiling from time to time, encouraging me to sit in silence a little longer or prompting me with a question for one of my frequent guests. This table at Borders wasn't much, but it was a space where I regularly experienced an embodied sense of Home.

But in the days and weeks after being unceremoniously fired, this table of goodness and fellowship increasingly became a table of loneliness and pain. A darkness seemed to hover. I sat in the same chair at the same table where I'd once laughed and even cried with dear friends, where I'd felt a deep sense of connection to Jesus—but now, all I felt was empty. I couldn't see the face of Jesus or hear his voice. I felt alone and very, very angry. It wasn't just that my calling was somehow undermined, but now even the safety of this table—the place I had fulfilled that calling most acutely—seemed compromised. For years I'd felt at home in my body in this sacred place; now I vigilantly scanned the store, terrified I might see a leader from church walking around.

I pulled my chair farther back in the corner. I'd been tugged out to sea, now mired in Storm. Tears streamed even as my anger seethed. The warning lights on my personal dashboard were so bright that they might've been seen from miles away. I knew I needed to find another place to sit with my pain.

I drove a few miles away to a retreat center where, tucked away in the trees, sat a chapel, often empty. I found my way to the altar of the chapel where, before three chairs in which I'd hoped to find the Father, Son, and Holy Spirit, I began to cry. My cries were angry ones, recalling the laments of Scripture:

Why, LORD, do you stand far off?
Why do you hide yourself in times of trouble?

PSALM 10:1

My soul is in deep anguish.
   How long, Lord, how long?

PSALM 6:3

My tears have been my food
   day and night,
while people say to me all day long,
   "Where is your God?" . . .
Your waves and breakers
   have swept over me.

PSALM 42:3, 7

You have put me in the lowest pit,
   in the darkest depths. , , ,
   Darkness is my closest friend.

PSALM 88:6, 18

My God, my God, why have you abandoned me?

MATTHEW 27:46, NLT

Waves of earlier traumatic encounters came back to me, memories of feeling cast out, cut off, unfairly treated, even bullied. My body surged with angry energy. I flailed my arms and kicked the air. "Where were you, God?" I cried.

I remembered a lament of C. S. Lewis that I'd shared many times in sermons and teachings:

But go to Him when your need is desperate, when all other help is vain, and what do you find? A door slammed in your face, and a sound of bolting and double bolting on the inside. After that, silence.[1]

The door had been slammed. I couldn't see or hear God. I felt only shame, abandonment, rejection. Silence.

It was too much.

So I cast these awful feelings into the shadows. While I don't think I realized I was doing this, I'd been thrust into a dark night of the soul, and I ran from it.

The Dark Night and Addiction

The language of the dark night was coined by a Spanish monk named St. John of the Cross, a man who taught and wrote around the same time as many sixteenth-century Protestant Reformers. A man not even five feet tall, St. John was neither imposing nor intimidating, but his honest calls for reform in the church got him into trouble. Like Martin Luther's, his protestations caught the attention of the dutiful guardians of church teaching and practice and landed him in a prison cell for nine months. In the dark and damp, all he could hear was the sound of his breath and the squealing of rats, who'd made his abode theirs. Overwhelmed and frightened, he faced the inevitable questions each of us face in our moments of powerlessness, fear, and loneliness.

It might have been a traumatizing time. All he'd counted as

stable in his life had been taken from him. His future, even his health and safety, was uncertain. It must have been utterly terrifying, awakening within him feelings of abandonment, uncertainty, and powerlessness. But he did something remarkable—he gazed into the darkness. He befriended it, along with all of the uncomfortable feelings that came with it. He refused to ignore what this season would teach him.

In that dreary cell, his old strategies would die. His smaller versions of God would fade. His futile attempts at control would be crushed. It was dark—pitch-black—so bleak that he couldn't see. But his eyes would eventually adjust, allowing him to reckon with everything he'd relegated to the shadows, allowing him to see God anew.

This dark night experience isn't as rare as you might think. Each of us encounters the dark night at some point in our journey. However, in our overstimulated and chronically busy lives, we often remain unaware of its presence, evading its revelation to us. If we did want to be aware of it, though, what might we keep an eye out for?

The dark night doesn't always appear as dramatically as it did for St. John of the Cross, even as suddenly as it did for me in the weeks after being fired. In fact, you may simply experience a dulled sense of God's comfort or presence. Joy and delight may begin to feel far away. You may notice that your everyday addictions, even your tried-and-true spiritual practices, aren't keeping your restlessness at bay as they once did. Worse still, for a time, even quite a long time, it may feel as if you're coming apart at the seams, as if everything you've found soothing or solace in is being torn from you. You may sense something lurking within, but you'll likely redouble your efforts to avoid it.

Yet, ask an addict in real sobriety about once and for all facing the pain he's tried to medicate away, and he'll likely tell a dark night story. He may not know about St. John of the Cross, but he'll easily tell you how he ran from what he was afraid lurked in the pitch-black, deep within. He'll tell you how he resisted facing what hid in the shadows. This is where addiction meets the dark night—addiction medicates that which is too painful to feel and too scary to look at within us.

But the gift of the dark night is that it dulls the enjoyment of our coping mechanisms, it robs our small-*g* gods of their power, it turns off the power to our self-satisfying salves. And some of these salves, we discover, are not the big, bad addictions we typically identify with those so-called problem people "out there" but the ones we've sanctified within the fold.

Addictions in Church Clothes

Unlike St. John of the Cross, I'd resist meeting God in the dark night for almost a decade.

It wasn't until I lay in agony in a hospital bed in Mexico that I truly turned toward what was happening within. I was far away from home, and far from myself too. As my body recovered in the weeks after my gallbladder surgery, I began to sense the toll that trauma from years earlier had taken. As I was running from my dark night, I had mustered up everything within me to provide for my family and to forge a way vocationally.

But while our addictions may keep the pain at bay for a season, a Storm battering us from within for months, if not years, takes a toll. It was now painfully obvious that I was paying the price: an ailing body, a weary soul, a short temper, buzzing anxiety, and a growing Fog of depression that frightened me.

How did I get here? How did it get this bad? The truth is, on the outside I looked like someone whose faith was sturdy and intact, but my addictions were just dressed in church clothes. Indeed, while there are addictive ways of coping with trauma that, on the surface, are terribly harmful to oneself and others, there are also religiously approved ways of coping—and they are extremely convincing covers for pain. I recall mentors of mine praising me for my so-called resilience, and I was feeling pretty proud about pulling myself up by my bootstraps. In fact, some of the best fig-leaved cover for trauma comes in the form of religious addiction, mired in images and analogies that don't serve mature spirituality. Seldom is someone "caught" in a religious addiction as they are in various other forms of addiction. Much of the time, it looks holy, devoted, and pure, as it did for me. It comes with praise and perks. But it's still an addiction, and it still operates from a place of deficit and disconnection. Many never awaken to their spiritually sanctioned ways of coping, even within a dark night.[2]

Consider a few stories that illustrate this. I knew a woman who lived what seemed like a faithful life to many, devotedly serving her family, dutifully submissive to her husband, according to her cherished belief. As a child she'd experienced significant trauma and learned early in life not to speak up, behavior that was ennobled as humility. She lived much of her adulthood in Fog, shut down to her emotions and resigned to her husband's humiliating forms of control. Her quiet anger would sometimes surface, particularly as she got older and as dementia stole her normal coping mechanisms. But as she and her husband celebrated their fiftieth anniversary with friends, giving gratitude to God for a faithful marriage, I couldn't help but feel a profound sadness amidst unrecognized trauma. This spiritually sanctioned style of coping had only sequestered her more painful emotions to the shadows, which kept her from being truly known.

Here's another story. A church planter wowed an assessment team I was working with, his presence strong and his gifts evident to the entire team. He preached a sermon that brought all of us to tears, and we sent him off to plant a new church with our blessing. Two years later, he called me with a surprise confession: He'd had an affair and was planning to leave his wife of ten years. "I'm not sure I ever believed any of this faith stuff anyway," he told me. Curious, I went to his church web page to listen to his sermon from just two days prior. It, too, was deep, beautiful, and eloquent. It even seemed heartfelt. Yet none of it was coming from his true heart of hearts; it was a smoke screen of deceit. My friend ended up trying to repair his marriage and rediscover faith, and that's when the real truth surfaced: Underneath the perfect image he had curated were stories of profound childhood pain that he'd never before shared with anyone, shame and abuse covered in shiny church clothes.

Finally, another woman I knew danced between church

committees, always cheery. Though she was often praised for her positivity, I sensed an underlying sadness that no one ever dared discuss with her. I'd heard rumors of multiple miscarriages and a challenging marriage, but the image she presented was what others called a "fervent faith," motivation for her to continue chugging along. That is, until a difficult diagnosis came. While she attempted to remain cheerful on her social media care page, she privately admitted to me that major questions about God's goodness and her worth stirred within. Gently, I asked if she could once and for all acknowledge the profound sadness and anger she'd medicated away through her religious addictions. She wanted to. But in the end, she had an image to maintain. She worried that her honesty would cause people to question God's goodness. People needed her to be cheery, even if it meant further suffering for her.

The spiritual theologian Karl Rahner offers an honest picture of what happens when we've become accustomed to—even feel entitled to—the things that have served us so well:

> If we think that God must be at our disposal as long as
> and because we serve him; if we think it isn't right that
> things should go badly; if this is how we think, then
> behind these cherished illusions there is a false image
> of God and this is what we serve. If these images are
> shattered by God himself and his life, by his guidance
> and providence, then one thing should be clear from
> the beginning: what is disappearing is not God, but
> an idol.[3]

St. John's dark night of the soul is a crucible in which any form of addiction can wither, but its special revelation is reserved for religious addictions, not least the myriad ways in which we embody the persona of a faithful follower of Jesus. What St. John realized in his cell was that his old idols, even the seemingly good things he'd wrapped his heart around, couldn't produce the life in him that he longed for. Amidst his captivity, he sensed an opening within, an interior freedom growing even as he remained bound. Despite what had happened to him, he became attuned to what was happening within himself. And what was happening within was a "complete undoing," but it was an undoing that would remake him.[4]

The gift of a dark night is this: Our cherished addictions— sometimes even the good practices we've come to depend on— lose their power to provide the soothing we need. It's as if the power source that once lit up our life of restless addiction is pulled, and the lights go out. Many find that long-held habits of prayer and worship don't elicit feelings of comfort or consolation like they used to. Some return to an old devotional book or a once-cherished worship song, hoping it might fan the flame of devotion, but the spark doesn't ignite. God is calling us to more, but we might not even know it. We may just redouble our efforts at self-soothing.

With some curiosity, maybe even with the wise aid of a spiritual director or contemplatively informed therapist, could we courageously allow ourselves to awaken to the gift of the dark night? True, it holds the possibility of a painful revelation, but it's one that may offer us the gift of ourselves and the gift of God in return. What we discover is that the dark we're running from might just be the very place where we can find God, where we can discover reunion and reconnection, where we're made whole again.

More than fifty years ago, the prolific author and renowned monk Thomas Merton described how we might face this dark night ourselves. He wrote that the dark night invites us to be "drawn out from behind our habitual and conscious defenses" that are designed to protect us from the "unconscious forces that are too great for us to face naked and without protection."[5] Merton's "habitual defenses" are our strategies for medicating the pain, our manifold addictions, even our addictions in church clothes. And the "unconscious forces" are often the feelings that are too hard to face, the needs too shameful to name. These forces lurk in the shadows within, revealed in our sense of shame and sadness, terror and powerlessness, rage and rejection, emptiness and abandonment. The dark night of the soul invites us to attend to all of it.

> If we set out into this darkness, we have to meet
> these inexorable forces. We will have to face fears and
> doubts. We will have to call into question the whole
> structure of our spiritual life. We will have to make a
> new evaluation of our motives for belief, for love, for
> self-commitment to the invisible God.[6]

In other words, we're in for a complete undoing. But one that may just save our lives.

Grace in the Darkness

"When you see that your desires are darkened, your inclinations dried up, and your faculties incapacitated," writes St. John of the Cross, "do not be disturbed. Consider it grace. God is freeing you from yourself."[7]

Of course, this doesn't feel like grace. And it most definitely is disturbing. But something about it is unquestionably true—we discover grace as our old ways of coping cease to deliver, as we come to see that we can no longer live alienated from ourselves.

The grace of being freed from yourself, as St. John puts it, is the grace of being freed from the old you, the you (or yous) you thought you were. The spiritual you. The special you. The savior you. The idealized you. The perfectionistic you. The achiever you. The brilliant you. The powerful you. The workaholic you. The responsible you. The hypervigilant you. All parts of you that worked hard to keep you afloat, to allow you to survive. But parts of you that have been living by the old lie of that slithering serpent—that you've got to go it on your own.

When I finally returned to ministry after being fired, it seemed that all that had been lost was being redeemed: reputation, belonging, security, authority, respect, insight, opportunity, purpose. I fed on what my new city of San Francisco had to offer, my appetite voracious. Quite literally, my body remembers the dopamine-inducing goodness of the city's best cuisine and how a sip of Blue Bottle Coffee would send my demons racing off. But my voracious hunger was also satisfied in the many affirmations I got when I spoke and taught. I finally felt included, not only sitting at the leadership table but also holding a respected voice within the church I served there.

"Where have you taken your hunger?" God asks. And our answer demands honesty, even when it seems things are going quite well. Because amidst the seeming goodness of it all, my gratitude was tempered by a growing sense of an inner emptiness and budding depression. I didn't expect it, particularly given how well my work was going. But I started to feel adrift, untethered, not myself. It made little sense. I was being given back things I'd coveted, and yet they left me with spiritual and emotional heartburn. Indeed, those parts of me that had helped me survive were running on fumes, and in my dark night I was being invited to surrender, to trust, to be known, to heal.

I couldn't see it at the time, though. I was still running from that chapel, from the unconscious forces and painful feelings that hid in the shadows. Landing in a Mexican hospital might have been the physical wake-up call I needed, but it was the force of agonizing disconnection within me, even amidst the good things San Francisco offered, that finally got my attention. While there were no gaping holes in me that anyone could see, hundreds of micro-holes had formed within the dam of my religiously addicted self. Those "inexorable forces" Merton hints at were pressing upon me, demanding to emerge from the shadows and be recognized. The night had finally gotten dark enough for me to see that I couldn't go it on my own anymore, that parts of me lurking in the shadows carried deep wounds that needed to be healed.

This, too, was a grace. The grace of my dark night. My clarifying night.

In moments like this, it's critical for these parts of us to know that it's safe to step back from their exhausting roles. But we can't negate the fact that this is a massive moment of vulnerability, a movement from control to surrender.

With the help of my therapist, I began to finally engage the workaholic part of me, the one who longed to provide for my family at all costs, the one who was addicted to being thought of as—and praised for being—strong, capable, and hardworking. This part had been in the driver's seat since my painful firing in 2003; when I finally secured a new ministry job, it only became more voracious because now it was terrified of losing what it had gained. It pushed harder, worked longer, and continued to neglect the basic needs of my body and soul.

But now I joined God in greeting this workaholic me with kindness and curiosity.

Hello, workaholic. Thanks for your efforts, but you must be exhausted.

He was weary, indeed. I asked him if he could step back from his role, but gripping fear emerged, worried that I'd make myself vulnerable again to being hurt and humiliated. This was a part of me that didn't want to trust God, a part that even hijacked the rest of me to assure my survival.

In an inner conversation, I thanked this workaholic part of me for striving on my behalf amidst the terror of being fired.

And I reassured him that I wanted to continue to work hard and needed his help. But this time, I'd set the boundaries and we'd do it in a healthier way. He did step back.

And I could feel an extraordinary internal shift. I felt myself again. Gravity pulled me down into my chair, and my spine lengthened. I took a deep breath.

I'd been gone for a long time, and though I'd navigated through the onerous, dark night, it felt good to be Home.

The Practice of Facing Your Shadow

Try this exercise on a sunny day. Find a sidewalk or a driveway in full view of the sun, and face it, your body's shadow cast behind you. And then walk ahead in the direction of the sun. Walk firmly, deliberately, as if you're large and in charge.

As you walk, pay attention to your face, the part of you a passing stranger may see. Notice how you present yourself to the world. Consider how you learned to walk the way you do and talk the way you do, how you learned to carry yourself and even greet others. Feel the energy of this front-facing you.

Now turn your gaze to your shadow. Notice its length, and how it follows you wherever you go. Begin to consider what parts of *you* you might have cast into the shadows at different points in your life. Consider the messages you received about the most valuable and welcomed parts of yourself—and the messages you received about the parts that might be better off tucked away. Notice, even still, that your shadow never stops accompanying you.

We've been on quite the journey together. When we began this book, we practiced coming home to ourselves. We began to understand the depth of our disconnection. We've come a long way since then. Now, we begin to see that there are dark nights in which our ordinary ways of coping are dulled and we're invited to surrender in love and trust. Now, our time together culminates in what Stephen Cope calls the "night sea journey":

> The "night sea journey" is the journey into the parts
> of ourselves that are split off, disavowed, unknown,
> unwanted, cast out, and exiled to the various
> subterranean worlds of consciousness. . . . The goal
> of this journey is to *reunite us with ourselves*. Such
> a homecoming can be surprisingly painful, even
> brutal. In order to undertake it, we must first agree
> to *exile nothing*.[8]

All you've learned thus far in the book in the practices of coming home to yourself, befriending your suffering, paying attention, redemptive remembering, saying hello, blessing what is known and unknown, and reading signposts come to this courageous fruition as you turn your face to the parts of you revealed in the dark, weary, and wounded parts of you that have suffered as you've gone it on your own.

Will God meet you here? It's a terrifying question to ask.

The lie of the serpent, of course, is that you're all alone. That you'll always be alone. That you're better off alone. The serpent's lie echoes within, a primal trauma whispering, "God can't be trusted. Go it on your own." If trauma is, indeed, not what happened to us but what happens within in the absence of a compassionate witness, if trauma is our aloneness with our pain, then it's risky, indeed, to consider abandoning our ways of self-medicating and waiting in the dark.

And yet we know now that we don't have to be afraid of the dark. Imprisoned in a rat-infested cell and longingly waiting, St. John of the Cross found himself reunited with Love. He wrote

O night, that guided me!
O night, sweeter than sunrise!
O night, that joined lover with Beloved!
Lover transformed in Beloved![9]

In a world of exhausting chases and cheap, self-help remedies, this is the ancient path that offers deep healing and transformation. But it can't be manufactured. When the lights go out, we're powerless. We may face parts of ourselves we've long forgotten, exiled away even in our youngest years. But here we also wait in expectation for the one who longs to "restore you to health and heal your wounds" (Jeremiah 30:17).

But perhaps God is calling you, too, to face the shadows. To stop, slow down, and sit in the dark. Maybe there your eyes will adjust to a dim light on the horizon, signaling the smile of the one who will never ever leave you or forsake you (Deuteronomy 31:8).

RESOURCES

- Iain Matthew, *The Impact of God: Soundings from St John of the Cross*
- Gerald G. May, *The Dark Night of the Soul: A Psychiatrist Explores the Connection between Darkness and Spiritual Growth*
- Barbara Brown Taylor, *Learning to Walk in the Dark*

Reflection

1. Are you familiar with St. John's language of the "dark night"? If so, how have you typically understood it? Many conflate this concept with depression, and yet it's something quite unique. Does it feel helpful to you? How would you articulate your own experience of it?

2. As you consider the parts of you that you'd rather have people see and experience, how would you describe this "you"? How has this "you" worked for you over the years? Why do you suppose this "you" emerged in the first place?

3. As you consider the parts of you relegated to the shadows, take a few minutes to simply ponder what it feels like to become curious about these parts of yourself in the first place. Is it scary? Overwhelming? Might it feel safer to put this work aside until you can engage this question with a therapist?

4. If you feel safe and comfortable enough to begin exploring in the shadows, what do you see? What parts of you
   were relegated to these places? Do you have a sense of
   why this was? And when? Try to focus on one aspect or
   part of you or your experience and see what you learn.

Practice: Facing Your Shadow

Creating safety

The most vulnerable parts of ourselves and our story won't
emerge from the shadows until we feel safe. They respond not
to coercion but to compassionate presence. This may be your
own curious and compassionate presence, or it may mean the
presence of a friend or a therapist. It's very important that you
assess the kinds of conditions in which you feel most safe for
this inner work. Before you begin, verify the safety of both your
external environment and your internal space. For example,
if you're in Storm internally, you'll need to engage whatever
resources you need to find your way back Home. Many of us
received mixed and confusing messages about safety at an
early age, so it's important for you as an adult to discern what
external and internal safety feel like for you.

An imaginative conversation

If it feels safe enough and if it seems like there is some room
and even some permission within you to get curious about
parts of you relegated to the shadows, you're ready to begin.
Open yourself up to an inner, imaginative conversation with a

part of you that might just feel much younger and much more vulnerable. Maybe it's a sad you that you hide behind an exterior of optimism. Maybe it's an ashamed you that never, ever felt good enough. Maybe it's an angry you that was never given permission to say no. You can use the parts exercise in chapter 5 (see page 127) to become a bit more curious. See what feelings, beliefs, or burdens this part of you carries, and consider what needs it might have. It's also important to discern how it might be cared for by Jesus. If this part of you could ask for anything from him, what would it be?

HOLY HUNGER

Longing to Be Found, Learning to Flourish

*Alienation and trauma of place are best met not with
dislocation but with belonging, with a defiant rootedness,
even if those roots stretch out to new and safer places.*

COLE ARTHUR RILEY

THROUGH MY VIRTUAL PORTAL ON ZOOM, I watched my niece, a wide smile across her face, walk the stage to receive her diploma. It was a familiar space, the same Long Island, New York, elementary school auditorium where I watched *The Little Rascals*, *Chitty Chitty Bang Bang*, and *The Love Bug* when recess was rained out. The same stage where I played my first band concert. Though grateful for the technology to allow me to peer in from Michigan, I felt a long way from the real thing.

I watched the likes grow on my sister's Facebook post of the occasion, old familiar names popping up like ghosts from my past. It struck me that my sister still regularly sees people we graduated with decades ago. Her girls get to hear stories about her MVP basketball, softball, and volleyball seasons from people who actually played with her. She regularly sees cousins whom I haven't seen in years, if not decades. And in minutes, she'd have an army of people flock to her family's aid in a time of need.

I transferred away from a local college on Long Island during my sophomore year, never to return except for summers and breaks. I met my wife, Sara, in Iowa, and we spent two years in Chicago, fourteen in Orlando, and five in San Francisco before moving to West Michigan, where we've lived ever since. My older daughter has lived in seven different houses with us; my younger, six. They've endured two cross-country moves. We even left behind my parents in Orlando when we transitioned away, a significant loss for my girls. I've wondered at times: *Where will they ever call home?*

We chalked all of this up to a transitional life in ministry, but we didn't count the cost decades ago. And while I'm proud of how my girls have adapted, I can't help but envy my sister's choice to stay, to send her kids to Sycamore Avenue Elementary School, to have the chance run-in with a familiar face at the grocery store.

The reality is, disconnection is a growing reality for most in the West. Though we live under the pretense that we're more connected than ever, virtually tethered through technologies like Zoom, FaceTime, and social media, we're lonelier than ever. Some call it a public health crisis, linked to depression, anxiety, premature mortality, decreased cardiovascular health, increased inflammation, and disruptions in hormones and sleep.[1] And the sad fact is that many, like my family, don't have the built-in resources of long-term relationships within the community to provide us support. We're literally doing it on our own.

Today many people are driven less by the need for community and more by career and competition, as Dr. Vivek Murthy, the US surgeon general under President Joe Biden, observes:

> Our twenty-first-century world demands that we focus
> on pursuits that seem to be in constant competition
> for our time, attention, energy, and commitment.
> Many of these pursuits are themselves competitions.
> We compete for jobs and status. We compete over
> possessions, money, and reputation. We strive to stay
> afloat and to get ahead. Meanwhile, the relationships
> we claim to prize often get neglected in the chase.[2]

I get it—the allure of adventure often overcomes the simplicity of staying put. The thrill of the climb might just be more satisfying than the slow, predictable cadence of community. But we might need to be honest about the losses we're incurring.

At one point when asked about our many moves, I brushed aside the losses. "We're kind of built for it," I said. So you can imagine how challenging these words from Cole Arthur Riley were to read:

> You make bravado out of your loneliness. It is one way
> to numb the pain of the wound. You elevate yourself
> above community, looking down at it as frivolous or
> needy or less enlightened—this is in denial of your
> own needs, of course. Both of these responses must be
> dismantled delicately, for underneath is the wound of

not being embraced or known or cared for well by those whom you have longed to know and care for you.[3]

Indeed, for as much as we're learning about the fundamental need for connection from the womb to our last moments of breath, we're suffering the painful effects of chronic disconnection as a society. And it's manifesting in all manner of mental health challenges, addiction, chronic illness, and more.

There is also a corresponding consequence. Amidst our disconnection, we're suffering—personally and collectively—from a deficit of desire. What I mean is that we're settling too easily, living too half-heartedly, compromising for cheap dopamine hits rather than the goodness, intimacy, joy, worth, belonging, and purpose for which we were designed. We're more and more apt to live comfortably disconnected rather than yearn for more.

God asks, "Have you eaten from the tree?" And as we've seen, his words invite us to ponder "Where have you taken your hunger?" That's a good and important question, one worth spending unhurried time considering. But there is a second question revealed if we listen even more closely. And it's just as important. Together, we'll spend the last pages contemplating it.

The question is this: What do you long for?

The Deeper Desire

It seems silly to write in a serious book, but I felt like the restless pangs and simmering anger of an addict in withdrawal one evening when HBO Max didn't give me access to a show that

I, and most of America, was waiting to watch. I was ready, drink and snack in hand, my body awaiting its Sunday evening soothing. But I turned on my television to find an error code. And it persisted.

I took a picture of the message and sent it to my family for sympathy, but they didn't respond. So I went to Twitter. Luckily, others were as aggrieved as I was. I took some solace in that, but I didn't dare share my own rage, as I didn't want to tarnish my reputation as a wise contributor to social media. After all, it was just a TV show.

Except the error code kept blinking. More time elapsed, and while I continued to reset my television, check my phone, and nurse my agitation, I quietly resented my family's lack of concern. So, I clicked the question mark reaction on our family text thread to get their attention. They still didn't respond. You might surmise that I took the next few minutes to meditate or practice contemplative prayer of some kind, reconnecting to myself and to God.

I most certainly did not.

Instead, I stewed, refreshing both Twitter and HBO Max with frenzy, my body now feeling the full effects of withdrawal. My daughter texted, "What's up?" I wanted to respond, "Only the end of the world!" But then, by God's grace, the magic elixir appeared, the error code gone and the portal to my beloved show opened up. The screen produced a soothing chemical cocktail within me, and I sighed deeply. I felt okay again.

The twenty-first century has given us more ways to feel comfortably numb than we've ever had before. If you want to know whether you're addicted, ask yourself how alive you feel on any given day, or how deeply you long for goodness, truth, and beauty. Addiction dulls us to beauty. Ask yourself if your heart is stirred by a flock of geese flying overhead, or the giggle of a wide-eyed baby. Ask yourself if your heart still skips a beat when you look at your spouse of thirty years or when you catch a rare glimpse of a pileated woodpecker. Hearts that are alive and full of longing don't often settle for cheap elixirs.

Truth is, I'm probably not going to give up watching TV altogether. But the incident reminded me of how easily a seemingly benign custom can numb and clog the spaces of our souls where love and longing are meant to flow freely. God's third question leads us to ask, "Where have you taken your hunger?" We've taken our hunger to hours of mindless scrolling, battles with social media foes, and binges of the latest shows. We may or may not have a problem with abusing substances, paying for sex, or gambling away our retirement. As we've seen, our addictions may be culturally approved or spiritually sanctioned, like the workaholism and perfectionism so many live with. No matter, they still suck the life out of us.

Where we go with our hunger is a good and important question, one worth spending unhurried time considering. But I wonder if that, too, is a signpost, leading us to go even deeper—to consider what is driving that hunger in the first place.

What do you long for?

That life that is sucked out of you—your God-breathed desire—is your longing. It is what makes you human. Gerald G. May writes,

There is a desire within each of us, in the deep center of ourselves that we call our heart. We were born with it, it is never completely satisfied, and it never dies. We are often unaware of it, but it is always awake. It is the human desire for love. Every person on this earth yearns to love, to be loved, to know love. Our true identity, our reason for being, is to be found in this desire.[4]

May is echoing what we've learned from both attachment theorists and ancient wisdom. We're born in and for love. Desire is that deep-and-wide river of love within you. Your self-soothing strategies are desire substitutes. "Addiction exists wherever persons are internally compelled to give energy to things that are not their true desires," May says. It "sidetracks and eclipses the energy of our deepest, truest desire for love and goodness."[5] These compulsions live in the gap where longing and love should grow and blossom.

And this is precisely where Jesus meets us.

The Compassion of Vulnerability

On almost every page of the Gospel accounts, we come across some version of this question of longing: *What do you want? What are you hungry for? What are you thirsting after?*

Time and again, Jesus invites people just like you and me to hunger and thirst more deeply. After all, among the first words of Jesus' most famous sermon we hear, "Blessed are those who hunger and thirst" (Matthew 5:6).

Alongside a well named for Jacob, the patriarch who walked with a limp, Jesus meets a woman who is thirsty. He says to her, "Everyone who drinks this water will be thirsty again, but whoever drinks the water I give them will never thirst. Indeed, the water I give them will become in them a spring of water welling up to eternal life" (John 4:13-14). The woman, we're told, is a Samaritan, which is to say she is an outcast, a member of a group known for bad blood, bad behavior, and bad theology. But Jesus doesn't slice the world into outsiders and insiders, bad guys and good guys, the addicts and the abstinent. At the well of Jacob, Jesus compassionately greets a woman who is thirsty, a woman created in his image, longing for worth, belonging, and purpose at her core. He doesn't mock her thirst. He doesn't shame her actions or her identity. Like Jacob many centuries earlier, she sees God face-to-face and walks away with a blessing. She arrives an outcast and leaves at peace with God and herself. She then encourages others to drink from his deep well.

When Jesus invites us to hunger and thirst more deeply, he always leads with compassion. Writing a century after Jesus, St. Irenaeus of Lyons makes the observation that God "does not use violent means to obtain what He desires."[6] With compassion, Jesus greets tax collectors, prostitutes, orphans, widows, and the diseased with some form of the question, "What do you want?"

He greets you with that question—and that compassion—too.

Compassion. It's a word that literally means "with-suffering." In Greek it is *splagchnizomai*, a word used to describe how one is moved to the core, stirred in the depths of one's spirit. It's central to the paradigmatic parable of God's lavish love and extraordinary grace. As Jesus said, "But while he was still a long way off, his father saw him and was filled with compassion for him; he ran to his son, threw his arms around him and kissed him" (Luke 15:20). And it's this compassion that tenderized the guarded heart of the young prodigal.

I'm convinced that it's God's compassion that creates the safety we need in order to long for more. Trauma shuts the gates of desire. Wounds wall us off to the love we need. When we don't feel safe, we'll do anything we can to protect ourselves. It's hard to long for more when we're guarded, when we've become invulnerable, when we don't allow ourselves to be moved to the core and stirred to the depths.

C. S. Lewis's oft-quoted passage from *The Four Loves* seems apt:

> To love at all is to be vulnerable. Love anything, and
> your heart will certainly be wrung and possibly be
> broken. If you want to make sure of keeping it intact,
> you must give your heart to no one, not even to an
> animal. Wrap it carefully round with hobbies and
> little luxuries; avoid all entanglements; lock it up safe
> in the casket or coffin of your selfishness. But in that
> casket—safe, dark, motionless, airless—it will change.
> It will not be broken; it will become unbreakable,
> impenetrable, irredeemable.[7]

Our fig-leaved strategies served us for a season, protecting our tender hearts. But the longer we remain here, the more impenetrable we become. We don't want our hearts to be broken again, do we? The serpent in the Garden was the first to break a human heart, its lie mocking God's trustworthiness, even eroding humanity's deep sense of satisfaction in God. Ever since, we've operated with suspicion, defaulted to survival, remedied our disconnection with self-soothing. Returning to the story of the Prodigal Son, we see that even the young prodigal moves to guard his heart upon approaching home; he quickly proposes a deal to become a hired hand if he is allowed to stay, a conditional belonging.

The scandal of the parable is that the father longs to give the son his image-bearing identity back, to return him to himself. The father never resigns, never quits, never dams up his deep well of desire. Indeed, the scandal of the parable is the father's compassionate longing for his son's wholeness and flourishing. And it's scandalous precisely because, in that compassionate stance, the father himself becomes vulnerable.

In fact, no first-century father would have brought shame on himself by running toward a child who'd disavowed sonship. Only a mother would have, one whose tenderhearted compassion would have been expected.[8] But the parable shows the father quite literally racing toward his young son, likely inciting the mocking glances of onlookers. He willingly absorbs the shame his young son would inevitably be subject to, all in order to reconnect with him.

Even when we resist opening our hearts in a posture of vulnerability, God risks everything to open his own, to meet us right where we are.

Yes, God is vulnerable. The word *vulnerable* comes from the Latin *vulnerare*, indicating a capacity to be wounded. While we distract, numb, cope, soothe, avoid, and resist, God moves toward us in compassion, first in the Garden, then in vulnerable human flesh. The word *trauma* in the Greek and *vulnerability* in the Latin converge on the word *wound*. It might not be a coincidence. God meets us in our wounds because God knows, in the flesh, what it means to be wounded. God's deep desire for us meant that he'd be willingly wounded in the process of returning us to ourselves.

As Brené Brown writes, the path to wholeness requires "excruciating vulnerability. This idea [that] in order for connection to happen, we have to allow ourselves to be seen, really seen."[9] Excruciating vulnerability. That sounds like a terrifying path for many of us. But the good news, quite literally, is that it's a risk God takes first.

The word *excruciating* comes from the Latin *ex cruciatus*, or "out of the cross." It was a word the Romans created because no other word could capture the harrowing experience of crucifixion. It strikes me as powerfully important for those of us trying to find courage to take this journey that God knows excruciating vulnerability. That God knows powerlessness. That God felt abandoned. That God took on flesh and suffered, even to the point of death. "Unless we frankly recognize that Christ's birth and resurrection come forth from places of hopelessness and helplessness," theologian J. Todd Billings writes, "we've not understood their meaning."[10]

Indeed, in this solidarity with Jesus, we're made whole again.

That's because trauma is healed when in our vulnerability we meet God in his vulnerability, arms stretched wide open in a compassionate embrace, even from the Cross. He enters into the Storms in order to bring peace. His deep desire for us unleashes our new longing for flourishing. His compassionate pursuit gathers every wounded and weary part of us into unity and wholeness. Hold an image of God's motherly longing to greet every lost prodigal within us and among us as you read the words of the eleventh-century archbishop St. Anselm of Canterbury: "Jesus, as a mother you gather your people to you: You are gentle with us as a mother with her children."[11]

God is wounded so that our wounds might be healed. God's deep desire for our healing and wholeness unleashes our deep desire for it. God's compassionate vulnerability unleashes our capacity for compassionate vulnerability.

The Slow Work

If I'm honest, the question God asks scares me. "What do you long for?" Do I even dare long for more? Do you? With hearts prone to be broken, shouldn't we just "lock it up safe," as Lewis wrote, wrapping it round with anything that keeps us busy enough to avoid heartache? Daily, I ask myself, *Wouldn't I be better off on my own?* I'll be honest—I come back often to Cole Arthur Riley's words: "You make bravado out of your loneliness. It is one way to numb the pain of the wound."[12] These words haunt me because they're devastatingly true—of me and of so many I know.

Indeed, I lived there for many years. However, following the hard decision to leave San Francisco for a simpler, more grounded life in Michigan, I slowly discovered a growing capacity to be vulnerable.

Gradually, I allowed my heart to feel the sadness of years dominated by grasping and chasing. I grieved the choices I'd made that only bypassed my wounds. I allowed myself to experience God's longing gaze, his kind questions, his curious and compassionate invitation to hunger and thirst for more. I felt the vulnerability of it all—the risk to long again, to trust again, to hope again. Slowly, the Fog lifted, my nervous system soothed, and I began to live more freely, more intentionally, more attuned to previously ignored needs and disowned desires.

This vulnerability manifested in real changes in my way of living too. In fits and starts I attended more carefully to what I ate and drank. I began to exercise regularly. I wouldn't open my laptop after 5 p.m., a positively apocalyptic development for me and a shock to my family. I prioritized being available to my daughters, who'd become too familiar with my dissociative gaze. I discovered that my heart still leapt for Sara, almost three decades in.

I'd lived for too long in Storm and Fog, and I was returning Home. I'd spend more time here consistently. To be sure, I'd be tugged again and again back out to sea. The waves of generational trauma collapse on our shores and sweep us into the churn. Painful memories hijack the present moment. We become activated and agitated. But as we live here in Home longer and longer, our neural circuitry adapts, our body adjusts, and soon we're anchored for extended periods of time. We breathe more freely. We long more deeply. We realize that a life of flourishing actually feels pretty good. We risk desiring more and more of it.

We might even get a taste of the goodness the apostle Paul encountered when he wrote, "All of us! Nothing between us and God, our faces shining with the brightness of his face. And so we are transfigured much like the Messiah, our lives gradually becoming brighter and more beautiful as God enters our lives and we become like him" (2 Corinthians 3:18, MSG).

Found

I began this book with a story of discovering just how lost I was in a time that I'd hoped would feel like a Hollywood comeback story. I was in Fog after years of navigating a Storm of churning anxiety, trauma sparked by the humiliating experience of being fired. I'd been given another chance in ministry, and it was going quite well. But I sought in it Home on my terms, and I expected to find worth, belonging, and purpose through my exhausting labor. Work and ministry had become my addiction, providing welcome relief from the pain of facing myself in my shame, emptiness, anxiety, and anger.

But whatever short-term relief it offered cost me in personal exhaustion and an increasing sense of alienation from myself and those I loved. Leaving San Francisco was really hard, but I sensed a new invitation, not just to make a home in West Michigan but to find myself "rooted and built up in him, strengthened in the faith" (Colossians 2:7), living in a safer, sturdier Home that God was building within me. I'd need to turn my attention from what happened to me to healing what was within me.

Years earlier, when I left that chapel in the woods, I ran from the struggle. I was lost. And I was looking for someone to blame. But after a long season of suffering alone in an enduring dark night, God was inviting me to come Home to myself, to befriend my suffering, and to pay attention to the story my body was trying to tell me. In God's kindness, I was invited to remember my story, to greet the strangers within me with a hearty hello, and to bless what I could know and even what would remain unknown. Perhaps more challenging, I was being called to explore the signposts of my addictions and to face what I'd find in the shadows. Previously I'd been lost in *fight* and *flight*, *fawn* and *find*, *freeze* and *fold*; now God was longing for me to be *found*, to finally come Home.

It strikes me as profound that when Jesus tells the story of the prodigal's return home, the father welcomes him with sandals, a robe, a ring, and a feast, not with a sermon. The father trusts the son's body to remember. He hugs him, he touches his tattered feet, he holds his hand as he places a ring on his finger, he wraps a robe around his strength-sapped body. How immensely soothing this must have been! The prodigal was home, but he could now come home to himself, renewed in reunion and reconnection.

Jesus told many stories of being lost and found, and your life is one of them. From the moment Adam and Eve ate from the tree, God's heart was tuned toward restoration and redemption. The very first story is itself a story of lost and found: God the pursuing father and we the fig-leaf-covered prodigals, met with compassion; God like a seamstress clothing anxiety and shame-riddled bodies. Frederick Buechner paints the picture:

> But then comes the end of the story, where God with his own hands makes them garments of skins and clothes them. It is the most moving part of the story. They can't go back, but they can go forward clothed in a new way—clothed, that is, not in the sense of having their old defenses again, behind which to hide who they are and what they have done, but in the sense of having a new understanding of who they are and a new strength to draw on for what lies before them to do now.[13]

God meets you right where you are, tending to soul and body. And even though you'll stray once again, like lost sheep sometimes do, there isn't a moment when God gives up.

Back in chapter 4, I told the story of storming anxiety within God's people, who didn't trust but who went back to their deepest addiction for help, looking to Egypt, not God, to rescue them. God offered a pathway of rest and repentance, quietness and trust (Isaiah 30:15), and their bodies continued to storm within, as they raced off in search of self-remedies.

Trauma stirred and addiction reared its head, and even still,
God didn't give up on them. Left alone and exposed, God met
them, saying:

> Yet the Lord longs to be gracious to you;
>> therefore he will rise up to show you compassion.
> For the Lord is a God of justice.
> Blessed are all who wait for him!
>
> ISAIAH 30:18

And just two chapters later, Isaiah offers news of God's palpable
care:

> My people will live in peaceful dwelling places,
>> in secure homes,
>> in undisturbed places of rest.
>
> ISAIAH 32:18

This is the story, time and again—God longs to bring you
Home.

"The story of Eden is not over, yet neither is it simply
repeating itself endlessly through history," writes Gerald G.
May. "Instead, it is going somewhere. I believe that humankind's ongoing struggle with addiction is preparing the ground
of perfect love."[14] I might add, humanity's ongoing struggle
with trauma is preparing the perfect ground for love. Often, it
takes us seeing just how lost we are before we long to be found.
It takes us counting the cost of disconnection before we long

for reunion and reconnection. And it takes the safe, compassionate, and unfailing pursuit of God for us to open our hearts to love again.

"Where are you?" God asks, inviting us to see just how lost, alone, and alienated we've become and encouraging us to come out of hiding.

"Who told you?" God wonders, inviting us to muse on the story of that original wound.

"Have you eaten from the tree?" God asks, inviting us to explore how we, through our own futile but fervent efforts, try to address the deep hunger of our hearts.

Let these questions be invitations, not vehicles of shame as you may have once been taught to hear them. God asks them all for the sake of restored relationship, reunion, and communion with him, with one another, and with a groaning creation, itself longing for restoration. This first story offers a foretaste of a God who will spare no expense to return us Home, even to the point of excruciating vulnerability. The question I continue to wrestle with is: How will I respond to his kindness?

Indeed, we're not fully Home yet. We're still navigating 1,185 chapters in-between, and I'm prone to forgetting the plotline. It's easy to fall back into my habitual forms of coping. Sometimes, self-soothing feels easier. Sometimes, I still believe myself to be too wounded to be redeemable, even lovable.

Shame's bite leaves a venom that stays in our systems for a long, long time. Even still, God knows it's a long journey Home. And he longs to resource us for the wilderness ahead.

Once lost, we're now found. We walk on with a new understanding and a new strength, empowered by a vulnerable God who makes the way for us. And each day is an opportunity to live in this light.

The Practice of Compassion and Curiosity

I know you can do this. You've been pulled out to sea, to be sure, tossed in the waves of Storm, stuck in the grip of thick Fog. But you've learned some things along the way. In these pages, in the sacred work you've done to come home to yourself, you've discovered that there are ways to attend to your body, to yourself, and to your story. With some holy hunger, you've come to discover not just your wounds but a deep longing for the goodness God has for you.

I couldn't be more proud.

There are mysteries to all of this that we need to honor. As you continue in this work, perhaps it's most important to know that it's not all on you. God began the pursuit long ago. And Jesus entered in with excruciating vulnerability, making a way for you to live in freedom, in wholeness, in connection. The Spirit dwells at the very center of your being, whispering words of love over you even amidst the continued lies of the slithering serpent. God has made a way. And now we walk in it.

In our lonely and disconnected world, women and men like you are needed to reflect God's heart for restoration and reunion. You who've attuned to healing what's within. You who've returned to yourself. You who are befriending your suffering. You who are redemptively remembering. You who are learning to say hello. You who are blessing what is known and unknown. You who are learning to read the signposts. You who are beginning to face the shadows.

Yes, you. You're walking a path too few walk. And I'm deeply grateful for it.

Because you've grown in courage, you now get to pursue. In reconnecting with your image-bearing worth, belonging, and purpose, you now get to exercise a holy longing for others. You now get to live as ambassadors of God's shalom. You now get to walk in the way of the one who saw Adam and Eve hiding behind fig leaves, naked and ashamed, and moved toward them with compassion, asking questions that opened them to consider the disorientation of their separation, the depths of their story, and the disordered ways of navigating their suffering. With your kind queries, you now get to awaken the homing beacon within each wounded, weary, and wandering soul you meet.

I'm not asking you to pretend you're a therapist or a spiritual director. I'm asking you to be you. Vulnerable you. Compassionate you. If you've slowly worked through the questions God asks, then you, too, will find questions for others. You'll be able to act as a faithful wilderness guide for their journey east of Eden. You won't have all the answers, but you'll know how to inquire from a posture of curiosity. And you'll certainly know from your story and mine that there is no need to be in a rush.

What you'll begin to see is that you're not the only one who numbs and distracts, avoids and ignores. Your heart may be moved, your eyes wet with tears, as you sit on the bus during your morning commute, aware of the allergy to silence and solitude, attuned to the alienation, alert to the squirming and scrolling that anxious bodies engage in. You'll be more apt to see how rushed so many are. You'll notice distant stares. You'll lament the resignation. Your heart will ache as, at a restaurant, you witness a couple sitting at dinner hardly aware of each other. You'll wonder, *What hidden wounds have led to such disconnection?*

"Where are you?" you'll ask. Maybe at first, people won't know what you're getting at. "Who told you?" you'll wonder, and with time, you'll begin to hear the confessions. "Where have you taken your hunger?" you'll invite, and you'll learn that they've been numbing for a decade, cutting to soothe, too depressed to even care. You won't know what to say or do. It's okay. Your compassionate presence is what matters. People long to be seen and known.

Despite the many ways people distract and numb, hiding behind fig leaves of their own making, you know their divine DNA. You know they've been made for image-bearing worth, belonging, and purpose. You know that beneath cheap chases and unsatisfying salves, their hearts ache with a holy hunger. You know that where trauma has chipped away at hope and trust, their hearts beat for God, for connection, for love. You can pursue them, knowing that you're simply participating in a work God has already begun. You're echoing the curiosity and compassion, the strength and vulnerability, of an immensely good God.

And so, with gratitude for going on this journey and growing in holy hunger, I'll leave you with a blessing, one God taught Moses to share with his priests as a word for wilderness wanderers like you and me, lonely and longing for the compassionate gaze of their kind God:

> The LORD bless you and keep you; the LORD make his face shine on you and be gracious to you; the LORD turn his face toward you and give you peace.
> NUMBERS 6:24-26

Remember this: God's heart is always ready to help you find your way Home.

RESOURCES

- David G. Benner, *Surrender to Love: Discovering the Heart of Christian Spirituality*
- Sharon A. Hersh, *The Last Addiction: Own Your Desire, Live beyond Recovery, Find Lasting Freedom*
- Henri Nouwen, *The Return of the Prodigal Son: A Story of Homecoming*

Reflection

1. What is it like for you to consider the question, "What do you long for?" How is it to hear that question from Jesus himself? As you think about this, pay attention to whether it's challenging for you to long for more. If so, when did your longings diminish?

2. Jesus makes a way for us through his own "excruciating vulnerability." What is it like to consider your own courageous journey in light of God's self-giving love in his life, suffering, death, and resurrection?

3. How does it feel to be invited to participate in this journey as one who calls others to attend to what's happening within them? What resources do you need for your own journey ahead? What unique gifts might you bring with you as an ambassador of God's shalom in the world?

Practice: Compassion and Curiosity

Living in longing

Take thirty minutes a day for the next month simply to hear Jesus asking, "What do you long for?" Notice ways you've dulled your longing through all manner of coping, and see what bubbles up from the depths of your heart for yourself, for those you love, for the church, even for those tough to love, bless, or forgive. Take time to write these longings down and share them with a trusted friend or counselor.

Practicing compassion and curiosity

Choose one or two people in your life, and see what it's like to pursue them with greater curiosity through the lens of the three questions we've explored. You're not called to fix, to solve, or to analyze, but simply to exercise your new muscles of curiosity and compassion. Try to live in growing awareness of how people live estranged from themselves, and what the cost is for that alienation and estrangement. See if you might grow in deeper longing for healing and wholeness more broadly, and allow your longing to become the centerpiece of your prayer, for yourself and for the world.

Acknowledgments

WRITING A BOOK MAY SEEM like a lonely enterprise, but most authors are accompanied by their own "cloud of witnesses" (and editors, designers, cheerleaders, and more!) who lighten the load and bring joy to the often arduous journey.

My cloud of witnesses begins with my wife, Sara, who by her presence creates the space in our home that allows the creative process to flow. When my life is noisy on the inside and the outside, Sara creates what the band The Chicks describes as the "easy silence," which offers that beautifully co-regulating calm and connection out of which the words flow. I love you, Sara.

To my now-adult daughters, Emma and Maggie: You inspire me. As I scanned my own story looking for fodder for this book, you were on every single page of it, even if your names don't show up here quite as frequently. Girls, your presence always brings light and joy and laughter. I thought about you two a lot as I wrote this book. And because you've both been psychology majors, I've loved our interactions about attachment, psychopathology, and so much more. I hope this book connects with you and reminds you of the Love that will never let you go. I love you both thiiiiiiiiiiiis much!

To Sam: You asked Emma to marry you as this book was being finished. And you gifted me with your own writing, so eloquently personal and vulnerable. I love your heart, your curiosity, and your honesty. Thanks for regularly asking me how the writing was going.

To Mom: You passed away before this book was born into the world. The grief is more pronounced because of our healing journey over these last years. I know you would have read this with curiosity and delight . . . and maybe even with a little hesitation. I can hear your Brooklyn accent even now— "Okay, sonny, what'd you have to say about your motha this time?" Thanks for being my most fervent cheerleader.

To Dad: You are an artist from way back as a graphic designer and more recently as a woodworker. Thinking about your careful craftsmanship, I slowed way down to write this book. Too often, I've been in a rush. But you were never in a hurry. I'd like to learn from you, to inhabit your slower way of being in the world more consistently. Even if you can't read this book today, I hope that somehow you'll hear my gratitude for your unhurried way.

To my sis: We've been through some kind of year. Kathy, we're so very different and yet you've always been a best friend and a confidant. Being with you in the days after Mom's passing was an immense gift. I know no one more fiercely committed to family than you, and I'm so grateful to call you my little sis.

To my beloved friends as well as my Western Theological Seminary colleagues, who encourage and show up, whether near or far, whether regularly or irregularly: There are too many names to mention, and I'd inevitably miss someone if I tried. In a year marked with some grief, I've been especially encouraged by your friendship. As someone who offers care, I've learned how to receive it just a bit better. And the intentional check-ins and notes have been especially kind.

To my agent, Don Gates: You've been an exceptionally thoughtful collaborator from the inception of this project. Your unique experiences and gifts offered much encouragement and fodder for improvement. I've never worked with an agent before, and I'm so grateful you took me on.

To the whole Tyndale publishing team, especially Jillian Schlossberg: Thank you for pursuing this book with such interest and intentionality. You have the special capacity to listen well and to steward a process that honors an author's work while being unafraid to ask good questions, push for more clarity, and even rearrange whole chapters in a way that serves the reader so much better. Your investment in your authors is sincere and authentic, and you've become someone I feel known and seen by. And to Kim Miller, whose careful editing and wise counsel improved the book in countless ways. Also to Lindsey Bergsma, Laura Cruise, Mary Campbell, Stephanie Abrassart, and Amanda Woods, thank you for your personal attention and investment in me and in this work.

And finally to God the Compassionate Witness: Thank you for running toward me, for holding me, for giving me sandals, a ring, and a robe, and for inviting me home for a feast. And for asking me these three questions when I was weary, wounded, and wandering, inviting me on a journey of healing what's within.

Notes

INTRODUCTION: THE BETTER STORY

1. Henri J. M. Nouwen, *With Open Hands* (Notre Dame, IN: Ave Maria Press, 1972), 50.
2. Peter A. Levine, *Healing Trauma Study Guide* (Boulder, CO: Sounds True, 1999), 5. See also https://www.somaticexperiencing.com/.
3. I first read of a "primal wound" in the writings of Richard Rohr. I later discovered earlier instances of its usage in two books, both called *The Primal Wound*, one written in 1997 by John Firman and Ann Gila and the second by Nancy Newton Verrier in 1993.
4. In a foreword written by Gabor Maté for Peter Levine, *In an Unspoken Voice* (Berkeley, CA: North Atlantic Books, 2010), loc. 150 of 6113, Kindle.
5. Anne Lamott explores the power of this one-word prayer in her book *Help, Thanks, Wow: The Three Essential Prayers* (New York: Riverhead Books, 2012).

CHAPTER 1: WHERE AM I?

1. Though the Enneagram is too often oversimplified or used as a quick fix, I do find it a useful tool, and I've written on it in various places. See, for example, "The Enneagram Issue: Reactive or Reflective?" *In All Things*, September 18, 2019, https://inallthings.org/the-enneagram-issue-reactive-or-reflective/. Sadly, it can sometimes be misused in ways that prompt us to spiritually and emotionally bypass real engagement with our suffering.
2. Sean Gladding, *The Story of God, The Story of Us: Getting Lost and Found in the Bible* (Downers Grove, IL: InterVarsity Press, 2010), 35.
3. Curt Thompson, *The Soul of Shame: Retelling the Stories We Believe About Ourselves* (Downers Grove, IL: InterVarsity Press, 2015), 86.

4. Some noteworthy resources: See Nonna Verna Harrison's *God's Many-Splendored Image*. On worth and dignity, see Richard L. Pratt's *Designed for Dignity*. On belonging, see Stanley Grenz's *The Social God and the Relational Self*. On purpose, see J. Richard Middleton's *The Liberating Image*.

5. "It is not the will of God, however, that we should forget the primeval dignity which he bestowed on our first parents—a dignity which may well stimulate us to the pursuit of goodness and justice." John Calvin, *Institutes of the Christian Religion*, book 2, chapter 1.

6. St. Augustine, *Confessions* (3.6.11), from *Nicene and Post-Nicene Fathers, First Series*, vol. 1. trans. J. G. Pilkington, ed. Philip Schaff (Buffalo, NY: Christian Literature Publishing Co., 1887), rev. and ed. Kevin Knight, New Advent, https://www.newadvent.org/fathers/110103.htm.

7. G. K. Chesterton, *Collected Works*, Volume 1 (San Francisco, CA: Ignatius Press, 1986), 35.

8. James Hollis, *The Middle Passage* (Toronto: Inner City Books, 1993), 99.

9. St. Augustine, *Of True Religion* (xxix, 72). As quoted in Charles Taylor, *Sources of the Self: The Making of the Modern Identity* (Cambridge, MA: Harvard University Press, 1989), 129.

10. Bernard of Clairvaux, *Honey and Salt: Selected Spiritual Writings of Bernard of Clairvaux*, ed. John F. Thornton and Susan B. Varenne (New York: Random House, 2007), 20.

11. St. Augustine, *Confessions*, book 5, chapter 2, from *Nicene and Post-Nicene Fathers, First Series*, vol. 1. trans. J. G. Pilkington, ed. Philip Schaff (Buffalo, NY: Christian Literature Publishing Co., 1887), rev. and ed. Kevin Knight, New Advent, https://www.newadvent.org/fathers/110105.htm.

12. John Flavel, *A Saint Indeed, or The Great Work of a Christian in Keeping the Heart in the Several Conditions of Life*, Christian Classics Ethereal Library, http://www.ccel.org/ccel/flavel/saintindeed.txt.

13. Ronald Rolheiser, *The Restless Heart* (New York: Doubleday, 2004), 120–121.

14. Gabor Maté, "The Wisdom of Trauma, Official Trailer," Science and Nonduality channel, July 19, 2020, YouTube video, 1:06, https://www.youtube.com/watch?v=70HNmSsJvVU&t=69s. Find the complete documentary at https://thewisdomoftrauma.com/.

CHAPTER 2: SUFFERING ALONE

1. Gabor Maté and Daniel Maté, *The Myth of Normal: Trauma, Illness, and Healing in a Toxic Culture* (New York: Avery, 2022), loc. 4553 of 12186, Kindle.

2. J. K. Rowling, John Tiffany, and Jack Thorne, *Harry Potter and the Cursed Child* (London: Pottermore Publishing, 2017), act 4, scene 4.

3. For a beautiful picture of *tov* community, particularly amidst contemporary issues of church abuse, see Scot McKnight and Laura Barringer's *Pivot: The Priorities, Practices, and Powers That Can Transform Your Church into a Tov Culture* (Carol Stream, IL: Tyndale, 2023).

4. See Daniel J. Siegel and Tina Payne Bryson, who talk about the importance of feeling safe, seen, soothed, and secure in their book *The Power of Showing Up: How Parental Presence Shapes Who Our Kids Become and How Their Brains Get Wired* (New York: Ballantine Books, 2020).

5. See Matthew D. Lieberman, *Social: Why Our Brains Are Wired to Connect* (New York: Crown, 2013).

6. Bonnie Badenoch, *The Heart of Trauma: Healing the Embodied Brain in the Context of Relationships* (New York: W. W. Norton & Company, 2018), loc. 649 of 6331, Kindle.

7. John Leland, "How Loneliness Is Damaging Our Health," *New York Times*, April 20, 2022, https://www.nytimes.com/2022/04/20/nyregion/loneliness-epidemic.html.

8. See Gabor Maté and Daniel Maté, *The Myth of Normal: Trauma, Illness, and Healing in a Toxic Culture* (New York: Avery, 2022), 293.

9. Peter A. Levine, *Healing Trauma* (Boulder, CO: Sounds True, 2008), 3–4.

10. Aundi Kolber, *Try Softer: A Fresh Approach to Move Us out of Anxiety, Stress, and Survival Mode—and Into a Life of Connection and Joy* (Carol Stream, IL: Tyndale, 2020), 34.

11. For more on this entire process, see Janina Fisher, *Transforming the Living Legacy of Trauma: A Workbook for Survivors and Therapists* (Eau Claire, WI: PESI Publishing, 2021).

12. Peter A. Levine quoted in Gabor Maté, *The Myth of Normal*, 24.

13. Peter A. Levine, "Video: Dr. Peter Levine on Working through a Personal Traumatic Experience," PsychAlive, https://www.psychalive.org/video-dr-peter-levine-on-working-through-personal-traumatic-experience/.

14. Quoted in Francis Weller, *The Wild Edge of Sorrow: Rituals of Renewal and the Sacred Work of Grief* (Berkeley: North Atlantic Books, 2015), 11.

15. As quoted by Bethany Dearborn Hiser in her book *From Burned Out to Beloved: Soul Care for Wounded Healers* (Downers Grove, IL: InterVarsity Press, 2020), 162.

16. See Kelly M. Kapic, *You're Only Human: How Your Limits Reflect God's Design and Why That's Good News* (Grand Rapids, MI: Brazos Press, 2022).

17. Francis Weller, *The Wild Edge of Sorrow*, 161–162.

18. Thomas Moore, "Come, Ye Disconsolate," 1816, first verse, https://www.hymnal.net/en/hymn/h/684.

19. "Psalms of Complaint—Study Guide," Yale Bible Study, https://yalebiblestudy.org/courses/psalms/lessons/psalms-of-complaint -study-guide/.

CHAPTER 3: THE BODY TELLS A STORY

1. Bessel van der Kolk, *The Body Keeps the Score: Brain, Mind, and Body in the Healing of Trauma* (New York: Penguin, 2014), 99.
2. For more tools on attending to thoughts, emotions, somatic experiences, and more, see the excellent work of Arielle Schwartz, *The Complex PTSD Treatment Manual: An Integrative, Mind-Body Approach to Trauma Recovery* (Eau Claire, WI: PESI Publishing, 2021).
3. For examples of others who identify weather patterns for the sake of spiritual growth, see Martin Laird's *Into the Silent Land* and Lisa Colón DeLay's *The Wild Land Within*.
4. These four *F*s are from the work of trauma and attachment psychotherapist Sarah Schlote at https://sarahschlote.com/.
5. See Jim Wilder and Ray Woolridge, *Escaping Enemy Mode: How Our Brains Unite or Divide Us* (Chicago: Moody Publishers, 2022).
6. Freeze is a kind of transitional state in between Storm and Fog, moving from sympathetic to dorsal, and you'll find it variously listed in different books and resources, sometimes called *hyperarousal* and at other times called *hypoarousal*. Regardless of where it is listed, I understand it as more of a hybrid state.
7. Daniel J. Siegel, *The Developing Mind: How Relationships and the Brain Interact to Shape Who We Are*, 3rd edition (New York: Guilford Press, 2020).
8. Frederick Buechner, *Telling Secrets* (San Francisco: HarperOne, 1991), 66.
9. Martin Laird, *Into the Silent Land: A Guide to the Christian Practice of Contemplation* (Oxford: Oxford University Press, 2007), loc. 64 of 2057, Kindle.
10. St. Teresa of Ávila, *The Interior Castle*, trans. Mirabai Starr (New York: Riverhead Books, 2003), loc. 700 of 3148, Kindle.
11. For a compelling look into the psalms and their invitation to us to find ourselves in God's story, see Kevin Adams, *150: Finding Your Story in the Psalms* (Grand Rapids, MI: Square Inch, 2011).
12. Diana Gruver, "Charles Spurgeon Knew It Was Possible to Be Faithful and Depressed," *Christianity Today*, February 26, 2021, https://www .christianitytoday.com/ct/2021/february-web-only/diana-gruver -companions-darkness-spurgeon-depression.html.
13. Hillary L. McBride, *The Wisdom of Your Body: Finding Healing, Wholeness,*

and Connection through Embodied Living (Grand Rapids: Brazos Press, 2021), 46.

14. Mary Oliver, "Fireflies," *New and Selected Poems, vol. 2* (Boston: Beacon Press, 2007).

15. Cole Arthur Riley, *This Here Flesh: Spirituality, Liberation, and the Stories That Make Us* (New York: Convergent, 2022), loc. 241 of 2620, Kindle.

16. For a body scan you can easily access online, see "30 Minute Body Scan," Calm, https://www.youtube.com/watch?v=TPwHmaaaxLc.

17. See Arielle Schwartz's work at https://drarielleschwartz.com/therapeutic-yoga-classes-in-boulder/.

18. See Andy Puddicombe, "The Ministry of Mindful Walking," Headspace, https://www.headspace.com/articles/walk-into-a-mindful-moment.

19. McBride, *The Wisdom of Your Body*, 108.

CHAPTER 4: WHOSE VOICES DO WE HEAR?

1. See J. Alec Motyer, *Isaiah: An Introduction and Commentary* (Downers Grove, IL: InterVarsity Press, 1999), 194.

2. For more on these four needs, see Daniel J. Siegel and Tina Payne Bryson in *The Power of Showing Up: How Parental Presence Shapes Who Our Kids Become and How Their Brains Get Wired* (New York: Ballantine Books, 2020).

3. Todd W. Hall and M. Elizabeth Lewis Hall, *Relational Spirituality: A Psychological-Theological Paradigm for Transformation* (Downers Grove, IL: InterVarsity Press, 2021), 172.

4. Hall and Hall, *Relational Spirituality*, 142–143.

5. An exceptional resource on how we experience relationship with God through different attachment styles is Krispin Mayfield's *Attached to God: A Practical Guide to Deeper Spiritual Experience* (Grand Rapids, MI: Zondervan, 2022).

6. There are many extraordinary resources on attachment. In this chapter, I synthesize from a variety of sources. These include: Daniel J. Siegel's *Mindsight* and *The Neurobiology of "We": How Relationships, the Mind, and the Brain Interact to Shape Who We Are*; Diane Poole Heller's *The Power of Attachment: How to Create Deep and Lasting Intimate Relationships*; Todd W. Hall and M. Elizabeth Lewis Hall's *Relational Spirituality: A Psychological-Theological Paradigm for Transformation*. I also draw upon the good resources at "The Attachment Project" found at attachmentproject.com.

7. For more on sympathetic activation in preoccupied attachment, see Daniel Hill, *Affect Regulation Theory: A Clinical Model* (New York: W. W. Norton & Company, 2015).

8. Siegel, *Neurobiology of "We."*
9. Hill, *Affect Regulation Theory*, loc. 2676 of 4592, Kindle.
10. Hall and Hall, *Relational Spirituality*, 164.
11. See for example Jeffrey Guina, "The Talking Cure of Avoidant Personality Disorder: Remission through Earned-Secure Attachment," *American Journal of Psychotherapy* 70, no. 3 (2016): 233–250, https://doi.org/10.1176/appi .psychotherapy.2016.70.3.233.
12. See Hill, *Affect Regulation Theory*.
13. For more on the neuropsychology of self-harm, see Terri Apter, "The Self-Harming Brain," *Psychology Today*, January 6, 2020, https://www.psychologytoday.com/us/blog/domestic-intelligence /202001/the-self-harming-brain.
14. Daniel Siegel explores this concept in *The Developing Mind: How Relationships and the Brain Interact to Shape Who We Are*, 3rd ed. (New York: Guilford Press, 2020).
15. See Numbers 6:24-26.
16. See Romans 8:38-39.
17. See Psalm 103:8.
18. See Luke 15:31.
19. EMDR, or Eye Movement Desensitization and Reprocessing therapy, is a slow and structured work of engaging trauma. IFS, or Internal Family Systems therapy, invites people to explore the different parts of themselves that cope and carry burdens related to trauma. And there are other somatic, or body-focused, therapies that prioritize how the body holds traumatically frozen memories from the past in the present day.
20. Henri J. M. Nouwen, *Discernment: Reading the Signs of Daily Life* (New York: HarperCollins, 2013), 135.

CHAPTER 5: SAY HELLO

1. Disney Pixar, *Inside Out*, 2015, trailer, *"Inside Out | Meet The Little Voices Inside Your Head | Available on Digital HD, Blu-ray and DVD Now"* May 11, 2015, https://www.youtube.com/watch?v=KiCWU8SrbBU.
2. Quoted in Gabor Maté and Daniel Maté, *The Myth of Normal: Trauma, Illness, and Healing in a Toxic Culture* (New York: Avery, 2022), 23. This contention is further elaborated throughout Bessel van der Kolk, *The Body Keeps the Score: Brain, Mind, and Body in the Healing of Trauma* (New York: Penguin, 2014).
3. Janina Fisher, *Healing the Fragmented Selves of Trauma Survivors: Overcoming Internal Self-Alienation* (New York: Routledge, 2017), 5.
4. St. Augustine, *Confessions* XI.29.39, quoted from Henry Chadwick, trans.,

Saint Augustine: Confessions, Oxford World's Classics (Oxford, UK: Oxford University Press, 1991), 244.

5. Wendy Farley, *The Healing and Wounding of Desire: Weaving Heaven and Earth* (Louisville, KY: Westminster John Knox Press, 2005), 37–38.

6. St. Augustine, *Confessions* X.27, quoted from David Vincent Meconi, ed., *St. Augustine of Hippo, The Confessions* (San Francisco: Ignatius Press, 2012), 296.

7. Pádraig Ó Tuama, *In the Shelter: Finding a Home in the World* (Minneapolis, MN: Broadleaf, 2015), 11.

8. Ó Tuama, *In the Shelter*; see chapters 8 ("Hello to Change") and 10 ("Hello to Story").

9. Maté and Maté, *Myth of Normal*, 35. Italics in original.

10. Martin L. Smith, *A Season for the Spirit: Readings for the Days of Lent* (Cambridge, MA: Cowley, 2004), 35.

11. Thomas Merton, *Choosing to Love the World: On Contemplation* (Sydney: Read How You Want, 2008), italics in original.

12. Curt Thompson, *The Soul of Shame: Retelling the Stories We Believe about Ourselves* (Downers Grove, IL: InterVarsity Press, 2015), 125–126.

13. Henri J. M. Nouwen, *Life of the Beloved: Spiritual Living in a Secular World* (Pennsylvania: Crossroad Publishing, 2002), 33.

CHAPTER 6: HIDDEN ROOTS

1. John O'Donohue, *Anam Ċara: A Book of Celtic Wisdom* (New York: HarperCollins, 1997), 122–123.

2. O'Donohue, *Anam Ċara*, 81.

3. Aundi Kolber, *Try Softer* (Carol Stream, IL: Tyndale, 2020).

4. See Mark Wolynn, *It Didn't Start with You: How Inherited Family Trauma Shapes Who We Are and How to End the Cycle* (New York: Penguin, 2016). Wolynn also offers the broad landscape of research on epigenetics.

5. Resmaa Menakem, *My Grandmother's Hands* (Las Vegas: Central Recovery Press, 2017), loc. 1800 of 5388, Kindle.

6. John Firman and Ann Gila, *The Primal Wound: A Transpersonal View of Trauma, Addiction, and Growth* (New York: State University of New York Press, 1997), 2.

7. Children can awaken to the reality of death as early as the age of four. See Virginia Hughes, "When Do Kids Understand Death?" *National Geographic*, July 26, 2013, https://www.nationalgeographic.com/science /article/when-do-kids-understand-death.

8. James Finley, *Merton's Palace of Nowhere*, 25th anniversary ed. (Notre Dame, IN: Ave Maria Press, 1978), 30.

9. Born in the fourteenth century, she lived most of her life as an anchorite at St. Julian's Church, Norwich. She experienced a series of visions, later recording and revising them in the celebrated manuscript *Revelations of Divine Love.* Wendy's allusion refers to a line in the Thirteenth Revelation—"All shall be well, and all shall be well, and all manner of thing shall be well."

CHAPTER 7: ADDICTION AND GRACE

1. Dawn Elliott Kendall, Facebook post March 2, 2023 and therapist at SoulfulYou.Life
2. Quoted in Brent Curtis and John Eldredge, *The Sacred Romance: Drawing Closer to the Heart of God* (Nashville, TN: Thomas Nelson, 1997), 23.
3. From D. H. Lawrence, "Healing," in *The Rag and Bone Shop of the Heart: A Poetry Anthology,* ed. Robert Bly, James Hillman, and Michael Meade (New York: HarperCollins, 1993), 113.
4. Gabor Maté, *In the Realm of Hungry Ghosts: Close Encounters with Addiction* (Berkeley, CA: North Atlantic Books, 2008), 35.
5. Johann Hari, "Everything You Think You Know about Addiction Is Wrong," TEDGlobalLondon, June 2015, 14:18, https://www.ted.com/talks/johann_hari_everything_you_think_you_know_about_addiction_is_wrong.
6. Quoted in William T. Cavanaugh, *Being Consumed: Economics and Christian Desire* (Grand Rapids, MI: Eerdmans, 2008), 17.
7. Gabor Maté and Daniel Maté, *The Myth of Normal* (New York: Avery, 2022), 232.
8. St. Teresa of Ávila, *The Interior Castle,* trans. Mirabai Starr (New York: Penguin, 2003), loc. 1068 of 3148. Kindle.

CHAPTER 8: THE DARK NIGHT

1. C. S. Lewis, *A Grief Observed* (New York: HarperOne, 2017), 16–17.
2. Much of this is reflected in my book *When Narcissism Comes to Church: Healing Your Community from Emotional and Spiritual Abuse* (Downers Grove, IL: InterVarsity Press, 2020).
3. Karl Rahner, *The Content of Faith: The Best of Karl Rahner's Theological Writings* (New York: Crossroad Publishing, 1993), 212, archived May 16, 2017, at the Internet Archive, https://archive.org/details/ContentOfFaith TheBestOfKarlRahnerSTheoloRahnerKarlLehmannAlbertRaffeltHarveyD .Egan1.
4. St. John of the Cross, *Dark Night of the Soul,* trans. E. Allison Peers (Radford, VA: Wilder Publications, 2008), loc. 1115 of 2338, Kindle.

5. Thomas Merton, *Contemplative Prayer* (New York: Image Classics, 2009), loc. 1104 of 1824, Kindle.
6. Merton, *Contemplative Prayer*, loc. 1104 of 1824, Kindle.
7. St. John of the Cross, *Dark Night of the Soul*, trans. Mirabai Starr (New York: Penguin, 2002), loc. 1593 of 1953. Kindle.
8. Quoted in Bessel A. van der Kolk, *The Body Keeps the Score* (New York: Penguin, 2014), 125, first set of italics added; second set in original.
9. John of the Cross, *Dark Night of the Soul*, trans. Mirabai Starr (New York: Penguin, 2002), loc. 408 of 1953, Kindle.

CHAPTER 9: HOLY HUNGER

1. See Arthur C. Brooks, "How We Learned to Be Lonely," *Atlantic*, January 5, 2023, https://www.theatlantic.com/family/archive/2023/01/loneliness-solitude-pandemic-habit/672631/.
2. Vivek H. Murthy, *Together: The Healing Power of Human Connection in a Sometimes Lonely World* (New York: Harper Wave, 2020), 98.
3. Cole Arthur Riley, *This Here Flesh* (New York: Convergent, 2022), 77.
4. Gerald G. May, *The Awakened Heart* (New York: HarperCollins, 1991), loc. 67 of 3687. Kindle.
5. Gerald G. May, *Addiction and Grace* (New York: HarperCollins, 1998), 14.
6. St. Irenaeus, *Against Heresies*, book V, chapter 1, https://www.newadvent.org/fathers/0103501.htm.
7. C. S. Lewis, *The Four Loves* (New York: Harcourt, Brace & World, 1960), 169.
8. See Kenneth E. Bailey's *The Cross and the Prodigal* (Downers Grove, IL: InterVarsity Press, 2010).
9. Brené Brown, "Can We Gain Strength from Shame?" interview by Guy Raz, *TED Radio Hour*, NPR, March 11, 2013, https://www.npr.org/transcripts/174033560.
10. J. Todd Billings, *The End of the Christian Life: How Embracing Our Mortality Frees Us to Truly Live* (Grand Rapids, MI: Brazos, 2020), 187.
11. In the *Westminster Collection of Christian Prayers*, compiled by Dorothy M. Stewart (Louisville, KY: Westminster John Knox, 2002), 128.
12. Cole Arthur Riley, *This Here Flesh*, loc. 1027 of 2620, Kindle.
13. Frederick Buechner, *Whistling in the Dark* (San Francisco: HarperOne, 1993), 105–106.
14. May, *Addiction and Grace*, 12.

About the Author

CHUCK DeGROAT is a professor of pastoral care and Christian spirituality at Western Theological Seminary in Holland, Michigan, where he also serves as executive director of the clinical mental health counseling program. He is a licensed therapist, spiritual director, author, retreat leader speaker, and faculty member with the Soul Care Institute. As a therapist, he specializes in navigating issues of abuse and trauma, pastoral (and leadership) health, and doubt and dark nights on the faith journey. He trains clergy in handling issues of abuse and trauma, conducts pastor and planter assessments, and facilitates church consultations and investigations of abuse. Before transitioning to training and forming pastors, Chuck served as a pastor in Orlando and San Francisco. He and his wife, Sara, have two daughters.